Women Talk Sex

Edited by
Pearlie McNeill
Bea Freeman
Jenny Newman

Women Talk Sex

Autobiographical writing on
sex, sexuality and sexual identity

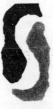

Scarlet Press

Published by Scarlet Press 1992
5 Montague Road, London E8 2HN

Collection copyright © Pearlie McNeill,
Bea Freeman and Jenny Newman 1992
The copyright of individual articles is held by
the contributors

The authors assert the moral right to be
identified as the authors of this work

British Library Cataloguing-in-Publication Data
A catalogue record for this book is available
from the British Library
ISBN 1 85727 000 2 pb
    1 85727 010 X hb

All rights reserved. No part of this publication
may be reproduced or transmitted in any form
or by any means, electronic or mechanical,
including photocopy, recording, or any
information storage and retrieval system,
without permission in writing from the
publisher

Typeset by Stanford DTP Services, Milton Keynes
Printed in Great Britain
by Billings Book Plan Ltd, Worcester

Contents

1 **Preface**
Pearlie McNeill, Bea Freeman, Jenny Newman

8 **Introduction: talking sex**
Patricia Duncker

15 **Going through changes for the better**
Bea Freeman

29 **Longings to have the blinds up and the light on**
Daisy McCauley

47 **No longer a victim**
Anji Watson

64 **Making sense of my memories**
Grace Walker

74 **Moving in, moving on**
Alice Land

83 **All about labels**
Halima

88 **… doin' it on my own**
Pearlie McNeill

103 **I'm saving up to leave my husband**
Kate Ashcroft

111 **Social security was the best husband I ever had**
Kate

121 **Taking the long way home**
Meg Coulson

142 **Confronting the angel**
Patricia Duncker

159	**Leading a life of my own** Jenny Newman
172	**Standing on divided ground** Celia Anwar
179	**Stepping out** Sal and Anne
192	**There's millions of the wee buggers ...** Catherine O'Shaughnessy
202	**The things my daughter taught me** Anna Moreton
210	**Bi–o–logical** Maggie Sansam
214	**Respect** B. J. Addison
223	**I want the world to shift on its axis** Marie McShea
232	**Acknowledgements**

Preface
Pearlie McNeill, Bea Freeman, Jenny Newman

The idea for this book was born out of women talking to each other. We knew that in the past there had been many attempts to define our sexuality, but none seemed to allow for the diversity of our experiences. From the beginning, our aim was to give each woman the chance to tell her story for herself, in a way likely to communicate with as many other women as possible. While we acknowledge that not every reader will find a mirror image of her own history, we hope that most will see points of correspondence. The more we hear other women speak, the more we realize that situations we once judged unusual are more frequent than we first thought. And even when our experiences differ, our conclusions can have a lot in common.

Society attaches a lot of importance to women as sexual partners, and not very much to the sexuality of individual women. And books purporting to be about women's sexuality sometimes end up being about men's sexuality instead. The prevailing myth would still have us believe that most people pair for life in monogamous, heterosexual couples, and stay happy that way, even though statistics tell a different story. Consequently, individuals who do not conform can feel isolated by a belief that no one is likely to understand their predicament.

For many of our contributors, revisiting the past in print has been an act of considerable bravery, especially when that past had once threatened to dam the powerful founts of creative and sexual energy which are rightfully ours. Hiding our feelings in order to conform to society's standards lowers our sense of self-worth and saps our emotional intelligence. It is being seen for what we are that brings us personal and political power. But not many of us make the journey towards liberation in one leap. Some women who have embarked on that journey decided en route that they did not yet feel ready to speak out. We have supported the right of any woman who wanted to withdraw her article, up to the very last moment, and the right of those contributors who wished to protect their privacy through the use of a pseudonym.

The word sexuality means more than just sexual orientation. Our understanding of it includes sensuality, eroticism, and the power to decide on the best form of expression for our sexual energy. As editors, reading each contributor's story has enriched that understanding more than any theory. Our joint aim has always been to share information in a spirit of co-operation instead of competition. Writing our own contributions has been an important part of this process.

Not every article here represents our own views. We made a commitment at the beginning to challenge unconscious racism or heterosexism in our contributors and in each other whenever we felt it was present. Otherwise, we always encouraged diverse approaches. An anthology can demonstrate the collective principle in print better than any other kind of book.

Many of our contributors would not call themselves writers. Some articles have been transcribed from tape recordings. Part of our purpose was to give an opportunity to women who might not otherwise get into print. Because so many publishing houses are based in London, there is a tendency for women living outside the capital to be ignored. As three editors committed to living in the north-west of England, we are particularly aware of this imbalance. And because the book trade is still dominated by white people, we have worked to ensure that one-third of our contributors are black. In the concluding part of this preface Bea Freeman explores the reasons why asking for contributions from black women is particularly important and challenging work for an editor.

This book does not attempt to present an overview. Nor is it a handbook. What we want most is for the book to generate discussion, and if other women go on pushing back the boundaries, then a major part of our purpose will have been achieved.

Pearlie

Sydney 1975. Over dinner amidst a large group of women, a friend tells me that she thinks I am a lesbian.

She did not mince words, but simply told me what she thought and why. Instantly I knew she was right. Something in me stilled that night as though every cell in my body heard those words and then relaxed quietly, breathing in the knowledge. Why hadn't I known sooner? Why had it been necessary for someone outside to reach in and tell me what I needed to know?

In the months and years that followed I returned again and again to these questions and many more. I began to ask other lesbians when they had known and how. I became fascinated by the unfolding of countless stories. Later, when conducting writing workshops about childhood experiences, women spoke of their teenage years: dressing up, experimentation with sex, using make-up and wearing high-heeled shoes that very first time. The trappings of femininity were more complicated than we'd been led to believe. I am still haunted by the story of one woman whose strapless ballgown stood alone on the bedroom floor, daunting its owner, who felt less female than the dress. Another woman remembered going home from boarding school with false fingernails, a tight skirt and lavishly applied make-up, in the belief that her family would be thrilled by this vision of budding womanhood. She was met at the station by shocked and furious parents and hurriedly bundled into a taxi as though she'd greeted them in her birthday suit.

I am still interested in the numerous ways we women have been indoctrinated, and in how we must first become aware of what that experience means to us before pulling away from the effects. I knew there was material for a book in all this, but the form remained elusive.

Then, in 1986, I attended a women writers' conference in Leicester. Noting that a workshop on erotic writing was on the programme, I went along. The facilitator was Jenny Newman. Before the workshop was over I'd written my first erotic story. Amazing. As I returned home after the conference my head was buzzing with ideas. I thought of a project, and mulled it over continuously. It would have to be an anthology, and I was sure I'd found the ideal person to work with me.

Would she be interested? I wrote a letter, addressing it to Jenny Newman via the conference collective. My excitement was growing. Impatiently, I waited for a reply.

Jenny
I was delighted to receive a letter from Pearlie McNeill, and felt enthusiastic about her suggestion straight away. The circumstances of our first meeting seemed like a good omen – a workshop of women who, without ever having met before, were all willing to discuss the complicated subject of women's erotic fantasies, and to go on to write a fantasy then and there, before reading it aloud.

I knew from facilitating women's sexuality workshops that trust and self-confidence and the readiness to share experiences are the best things to emerge from such situations. I also knew that there weren't many resources – books and articles – available to women wanting to find out more about their sexuality for themselves. Some of those on offer were written in inaccessible language, from an 'expert's' point of view, or else they catered for white, middle-class women, without ever conceding that this is a minority group. Here was an ideal opportunity – to produce a book that would reflect some of the experiences of the women I worked with. They themselves could contribute, if they wanted.

I have always seen myself as a reticent person, although I am convinced of the value of speaking out in print. I didn't know at first if my courage would carry me through an attempt to write honestly and directly about my own experiences, some of which were a secret even from my friends. But I soon realized that I would have to write an article myself before I could feel comfortable about asking other women to contribute. I was finding out that being an editor means more than inviting people to write. Contributors often needed encouragement and support while exploring their pasts. Like some of them, I still feel vulnerable about what I have put down on paper. A book does not remain the property of its authors. It has to take its chance in the world at large, and if it is to live at all, it will live in the minds of the women who pick it up from the shelves and open it.

Preface

Bea

When first approached to be a joint editor of this book I was taken aback. First, I do not see myself as a writer; second, I felt I did not have enough experience. Worried by questions about women and sexuality myself, I wondered how other black women would feel when I approached them. How was I going to convince them that their sexuality was a good thing to write about?

However, I took the bull by the horns, so to speak, and decided to accept the challenge. It was evident from the start that the two other editors knew the subject inside out and felt no embarrassment in talking about things I and other black women I knew would think too intimate for discussion, things that were personal, so personal you alone knew about them. What I saw as the other editors' confidence placed me in an awkward position. They knew I wasn't a writer, knew I hadn't covered the subject before, so why did they want me?

At one of our first meetings I asked this question straight out. They were open to discussion, making it clear that because they understood the importance of black contributors, it was a given in the situation that one of the editors be black. Nothing wrong with that, but would I have been asked if all the contributors had been white? One of the editors already had experience of working with black women writers and was aware of the sensitive issues that could arise. Both editors knew the importance of including black women's contributions in any anthology of women's writings. So I went ahead and approached a number of black women as possible contributors.

At first, they all agreed they would like to write something. However, once they knew the time for writing had come, some no longer wanted to contribute, or didn't feel it necessary any more, or couldn't manage to find the time. In some cases women began to write and then withdrew their articles. There were many reasons for this. For black women to write about sexuality and their personal experiences inevitably throws up many fears. Some women made the point that it was not sexuality but racism they should be writing about and, unlike some white women, they had never had the time to sit round discussing their sexuality. It is only recently that known black women writers have entered this arena, so the unknown writer can feel like a non-starter. The fear of exposure, laying ourselves open so nakedly, searching for the right language, these were the challenges. Could we meet them? Did we even want to?

Those women who did agree to write (and their decisions came about after lengthy personal debates) could see the value in it and wanted to convey their feelings to other black women who might have had similar experiences. The challenge was to share another identity, to make visible another aspect of our lives. For those who felt daunted by the prospect of putting their words on paper there was an alternative – they could talk about their experiences informally, using a tape recorder, and their words could be written up and shaped into an article at a later stage. This alternative was widened to include white women as well, and enabled voices that may not otherwise have been heard to be included.

Each contribution to this book presented by a black woman raises the question of racism, the thread that runs in and around the lives of all black women, and around our sexuality too. I found my editor's job a great struggle at times, and worried that I was not giving the necessary support to individual contributors, partly because sometimes other every-day things had to take priority. The point made early on about black women not having the time for projects such as this was as applicable to me as to many of the contributors. This was apparent at editorial meetings. White women's contributions always seemed to be in well ahead of the deadline, whereas black women's work was often late.

I found the discussions I had with contributors to be valuable in many, many ways, and I believe we all gained something from each other. It was wonderful to overcome our fear of sharing experiences that in some instances had never been spoken about before. When writing my own article I felt the exposure keenly and sometimes baulked at the process involved. But as time went on I was able to discuss my anxiety with other black women, and my fears lessened. We, the black women appearing in this book, through talking to each other and helping one another with as much care and awareness as possible, have transcended the seemingly insurmountable difficulties involved.

Our editors' meetings were lengthy affairs, but they were important because we all learned a great deal. At times I felt that I wanted to give up, simply because I was sure I had taken on more than I could cope with. As a black woman with untapped skills in this area, once or twice I felt tokenized. In any group there always appears to be a leader and I felt this happening, even though we made every effort to avoid it. I was aware of it, and at times I felt oppressed by it. This was partly due to my lack of confidence. But I did learn a lot, and as I was listened to and given more space to voice my opinions, suggestions and objections I could see that the other editors were learning too. We learned to trust, and to form a three-way friendship. Determined to make the project work, we took the risk and came to appreciate each others' strong points.

I would like to think that other black women would allow themselves to be open to the possibility of gaining new skills and knowledge, despite the obvious personal risks involved. Each experience must be taken on its own merits, and we must be as willing to talk about the positives as the negatives. Yes, there is a place for us as black women to come together with white women and share our personal experiences, and write about them. We can, black and white women alike, learn to network and struggle for change, and we can do this together.

I hope that this book, and the experience gained by the black contributors and myself, will spur black women on to further writing.

Introduction: talking sex
Patricia Duncker

Sex has always been notoriously difficult to talk about. In 1970, when I joined my first women's group with a confused idea that I needed liberating – although quite from what was still a mystery – we all wanted to talk about sex. And we couldn't.

Sex loomed large in the 1960s. We were convinced by the songs: *All you need is love*. And love meant a man in your bed. But we couldn't talk about sex comfortably, because we didn't have a language of our own in which to do so. So we talked about our relationships with men instead. In doing so, we were conforming to one of the central stereotypes about women: that we exist largely – only – in relation to others. The others being the men in our lives. We are his daughter, lover, girlfriend, mother, mistress, wife. I think now, looking back, that what we said was irrelevant. The most important step had been taken. We were women-only, amongst ourselves. We had closed the door and we were talking to each other.

Women Talk Sex has given me back some of the charged, infuriating, thrilling, frustrating emotional atmosphere of those first tellings, the emotional ear that listens critically but without judgment. Significantly, this book is based on the voice rather than on the written word; many of the contributions were taped. These are our words as oral history, as confession, as testimony.

I am very aware of the stories that are being told here that we didn't hear then. In my first women's group we were limited by our resemblances: we were all white, middle class and economically comfortable. We were too young and confused to decide what we wanted from our sexual lives, but we were the inheritors of the right to decide. In that we were exceptional. Very few women have ever had that privilege. *Women Talk Sex* presents a broader range of women's voices:

black and white, middle class and working class, lesbian and straight, women who could assume their right to decide on their sexuality and their lives and women who have had to fight to be who they are.

I listen now for the stories that I have never heard. I want to hear from women whose lives have been utterly different from mine, confident that in the recognition and respect of difference lies our greatest strength. Difference is not a simple matter, because it will always involve the uncomfortable realities of economic and social power, which while they remain unacknowledged can only cause division between us.

Within the women's liberation movement of the 1970s and 1980s sex and sexuality was the recurring item on our political agenda, as we tried to find new ways of talking sex as well as making love. Sexuality was one of our most disputed territories; it was the place where we have fought our most contentious battles. Our insight that sex was a private act with public consequences was the basis of our insight that the personal was indeed the political.

At first, in the 1970s, we believed that sexuality was something we ought to be able to shape and control in politically virtuous ways. If conventional heterosexual sex was oppressive and nasty, we would make him do it differently or throw him out. If we decided that men were a lost cause, we would choose women – each other – instead. We invented new concepts, like 'political lesbianism'. I remember having this carefully explained to me well over ten years ago now. 'It doesn't mean that you have to have sex with women,' she said, 'you just affirm your primary commitment to women. And you refuse to sleep with men.' It still sounds noble, but very mysterious. However, at last we were making the decisions. Many women did indeed decide to be lesbian: sometimes it worked and sometimes it didn't. The poetry, fiction and theory we wrote at that time, but above all the poetry, bears witness to our courage, joy, anxiety, rages, betrayals and emotional muddle.

The campaigns around pornography in the late 1970s and early 1980s transformed our understanding of sexual representation and sexual fantasy. Pornography was the most brutal skeleton in the heterosexual cupboard and the most controversial. Looking back, remembering our sense of menace and alarm at the depth and pervasiveness of sexual violence which we recognised in contemporary representations of sex and eroticism, I am not surprised at the sexual prescriptiveness that characterized many of our arguments and much of our writing at that time. The dust has not settled yet. The Great Lesbian Sado-Masochism Debate is still raging. Intriguingly, there has been no corresponding argument among feminist heterosexual women. Which saddens me, because a disinclination to argue always indicates surrender and defeat. No one could possibly pretend that all is well in the heterosexual garden, and many of the narratives in *Women Talk Sex* indicate just how unpleasant and difficult it is and has been there.

Sex is supposed to be the moment when we are most honestly, nakedly ourselves. This is a myth. Often we use the mask of intimacy to perpetrate the most destructive physical and emotional bullying. We use our bodies to avoid the issue. We exchange loving confidences in fraudulent currency. We fake it – again and again. We do this to hide, to deny our fears, to avoid honesty. We all live ironic lives.

Listening to other women over the past twenty years has led me to the conclusion that the problem of interpreting ourselves to ourselves is not so much how to tell the story, but which story to tell. I realise now that the story must be told again and again and again. And that while truth is multiple, many-layered, individual, lies are singular, definite, institutional.

> 'Women have always lied to each other.'
> 'Women have always whispered the truth to each other.'
> Both of these axioms are true.
> (Adrienne Rich, *Women and Honor: Some Notes on Lying*.)

Women's stories disrupt the conventional – that is the patriarchal – definitions of what constitutes truth and lies. Sometimes we need to tell our stories as fiction, ensuring that our left hand does not see what the right hand is doing. We use subterfuge, masks, disguises. These are the techniques of survival. And we have used them, above all, in our sexual lives.

I am very struck by the gaps, shifts, blanks in these texts. More than half the names attached to the writing in *Women Talk Sex* are pseudonyms. This has made me very uneasy; in what ways is this 'earthquake of honesty' compromised by the fact that we cannot speak publicly in the names within which we live. Here there are no easy answers. One contributor, wanting the whole truth out in the open after a life which appears to her as a pattern of hidden subterfuges and damaging lies, writes: 'I wanted the blinds up and the light on so that I could see out and others could see in.' Yet she is forced to write under a false name – which is the meaning of pseudonym – to protect others who have not been able to make that decision and who 'feel that their lives would be ruined were they identified with me.' In other cases, the women have been unable to write or speak their names for fear of their lives. There were several contributors who withdrew their narratives at the very last moment before this book went to press; women who did not feel safe, even hidden behind a pseudonym, with all the proper names and places changed. This is a terrifying reflection on the fear in which many of us live our lives.

But speaking the truth, even while your identity is masked, does not alter the fact that you are speaking the truth. Adrienne Rich comments on the urgency of the need to tell the truth in *Women and Honor:* 'When a woman tells the truth she is creating the possibility for more truth around her.' We become less fragile, less vulnerable, less intimidated by menacing silences.

Our writing about sex in the 1980s became more open, more encouraging, but still played safe. *Sex and Love: New Thoughts on Old Contradictions*, edited by Sue Cartledge and Joanna Ryan, was first published by The Women's Press in 1983. Imaginative and intelligent as that volume was, I remember feeling that we were holding our own experience at a distance, that our writing was barricaded around for protection by footnotes, the results of questionnaires, and academic citations. The exception was the joint contribution of two lesbian women who spoke about the problems of separation and dependency in their relationship. The disturbing omission was the issue of racism. None of the contributors dealt with the ways in which black women would have perceived the issues differently, or indeed how black perspectives would change the agenda. These were the new thoughts of white women, who were reproducing some of the old contradictions.

In 1986 I read one of the finest books by women on their lives, sex and sexuality that I have ever read, Sistren's *Lionheart Gal: Life Stories of Jamaican Women*. This too was a book based on the spoken word. Courageous and extraordinary, a band of working-class and middle-class black women revealed their lives, their struggles against poverty, sexual ignorance and deprivation – their moment in history. Racism takes a very different shape in post-colonial cultures; even when it is an inheritance from the white masters. None of Sistren have to live in what one black woman, speaking in *Women Talk Sex*, describes as 'a sea of hostile whiteness' where it is harder to trust others, harder to love yourself. Yet I would like to consider *Lionheart Gal* and *Women Talk Sex* as sister volumes: women's voices telling the stories of lives that have flowed underground, hidden, denied.

Women Talk Sex is a unique anthology not because it approaches new questions or new problems, but because of the way in which we have chosen – or dared – to speak. Here, we are thinking feelingly, interrogating our own lives rather than reflecting on generalities or hiding the uncomfortable embarrassment of our own hesitations, contradictions, confusions and muddles. Our own lives are our political, emotional material. A recurring theme in the anthology is the confidence and power felt by the women who have named, structured, controlled and possessed the raw muddle that is sexual feeling. Sex, sexuality and sexual identity have become interchangeable in this book. Sex is not only what you do, never mind who with, but how you feel about your body, what you choose to prioritise in your life and your existential grasp on who you are.

Similar, interlocking themes emerge from these voices. The ideologies that bind our joys and desires; marriage as the method of becoming respectable; our mothers telling us that sex is dirty, forbidden, taboo; taking responsibility for men's sexual urges, however uncontrollable, and taking the blame if we fail to control them. The darker threads are there too. I was struck by how carefully heterosexuality is policed, enforced by the patterns of heterosexual violence, child abuse, the systematic and casual assault of women by men. And by the fact that the lesbian women writing in the volume all had to negotiate all-pervasive heterosexual assumptions, both in their families and in themselves. Heterosexuality is the context for all other forms of human love. Never was the coerciveness of the entire institution more painfully visible than in this anthology.

Yet there are no stories about victims here. Again and again I charted the change in women. Our increased confidence in telling our stories, in freeing the needy, greedy, demanding child to become a woman who can take and give according to her own judgment and desire. There is an invisible revolution taking place in women's lives. It is as much economic as sexual. Controlling our own sexuality is about controlling our own labour, earning our own wages and spending them as we please.

Many of the women speaking in these pages are in their forties and fifties, looking back over the last thirty or forty years. I think that these will be remembered as the times in which our perception of our sexuality changed radically; that brief, momentous period of relatively accessible contraception for women before the advent of Aids. It is no longer possible, or responsible, to experiment sexually with the same freedom as this generation has done in the past. In *Women Talk Sex* mothers record the seriousness – and openness – of their sexual conversations with their children on the subject of Aids. We will have to find new forms of sexual expression, new ways of loving. And that may be no bad thing.

Sexuality can no longer be regarded as something fixed, immutable or unchanging. Our perceptions of desire are fluid, unstable, shifting. Many of the contributors use the metaphor of the voyage, the journey, the strangeness of ordinary lands. One woman, upon hearing her daughter declaring her decision to live as a lesbian, had the following reaction.

> I breathed a sigh of relief and thought thank goodness she at least knows where she's at – I'm still trying to find the map.

Even the labels attached to us by others are shifting, unstable, contradictory. One woman, reflecting on the pain and humour of racial labels, comments, '...first we were half-caste, then coloured, and now we are black.'

This book is filled with inventive, humorous refusals to give way, give up or give in. One black woman, taking imaginative revenge on her husband, decided to frighten him.

...he'd find suspicious motives in the things I said and did. On one occasion at least, though, I had a taste of sweet revenge. I called up the undertakers, told them my husband had died, and asked them to come for the body. I made sure that the time they were due was a time when he would be sure to open the door. If a black man could turn pale, he turned pale that night.

As I said, there are no women trapped as victims here. Many of these stories are narratives of escape.

Without the women's liberation movement, this book could never have been written. At its root are the principles we have evolved over years of argument and discussion; years littered with joy, dancing and pain. The editors decided to challenge any unconscious racism or heterosexism they sensed in our attitudes or their own. By doing this we are asking what kind of world we want to imagine or create; what kinds of women do we want to be? At least – and at last – we are asking those questions of ourselves, and amongst ourselves, across the inhibiting barriers of race and class. Not one of us ever fits the implausible stereotypes. As one of us says here:

> We black women have never been able to find ourselves in European images of women; growing up in Britain I didn't find any images of myself, nor could I identify with the few images of black women in the media or in my school books. So it was easy for me to understand that my white counterparts couldn't either.

Unsurprisingly, therefore, our sexual lives are diverse, unexpected, frequently violent and bizarre – we are often strangers to ourselves, to our lovers, our husbands, our children. Talking sex in the way that we have chosen to do here is to reach past the prescriptiveness of patriarchal systems with a good deal of laughter, anger and crying – to find each other.

This is, then, an emotional, difficult, peculiar and embarrassing book, full of strange courage. Wherever we live, whoever we are, it is very difficult for us, as women, to love ourselves. But this book is part of that difficult process, of asserting our right to love ourselves and each other, to be who we are.

Going through changes for the better
Bea Freeman

It has only been over the past four or five years that I have been able to look at and think about the words 'sex' and 'sexuality' and start analysing them in relation to myself. What do they mean? Did they have an effect on my childhood? How did I perceive them as a working-class child in the north-west going through my teenage years to womanhood? Most important of all, was my blackness tied up with my feelings about sex and sexuality?

As a child I knew boys were made differently from girls. I remember watching my brothers and a cousin peeing down a toilet together. I was very curious, and tried it out, only to find it was not possible. I also remember asking my mother why couldn't I pee like the boys? My mother was shocked to know that I'd been watching the boys in the toilet, and shouted at me. I knew something was wrong but didn't understand what it was. As I grew older I noticed changes, in particular that my brothers were no longer bathed with us. No explanation was given.

Just before my teenage years I went through a stage of wishing I was white. This came about because of games we used to play, like 'catch-the-girl kiss-the-girl'. I was never caught by the boys – it was always the white girls. I used to think that if I was white I would get that kiss and have a boy put his arms around me. I used to wish and wish that something would happen to me with one of the boys so that I could prove to my friends and myself that nothing was wrong with me. Even the black boys would only catch the white girls. In other games like 'dare', I would be the one to lift up my dress and show my knickers, only to be told off by adults if I got found out, which I so often did. I would hop over the black lines on the pavement, because the rule among girls was that if you stopped on these you would end up marrying a black man. I would always find myself jumping higher than the white girls.

My childhood fantasy was that I would fall in love with a white boy; that we would marry and my children would be white with blond straight hair, and that I would live in America. During my adolescence I would spend hours reading comics. My heroines were white women, cinema stars like Doris Day, Debbie Reynolds and Judy Garland. These images remained with me until late in my teens. Then I started to read women's magazines and the problem and letter pages over and over again. I found it amazing that women were writing about what I thought then were their most intimate problems, like periods and sexual intercourse.

I knew very little about sex and wanted to know what certain words meant, like 'masturbation', 'cervix', and 'clitoris'. I used to talk to my friends about what I had read, but they were vague about these issues and I found that I was not getting the information I required. My friends used to comment that all I wanted to talk about was sex, so trying to talk made me feel guilty, as if something was wrong with me.

All my close friends were white. They were convinced black people were different, and that as black boys grew older their penises were bigger than white men's. Although I tried very hard to dismiss questions and false accusations, they did make me think at times that sex and love were only for white people. I knew this was not true because my parents, my aunts and uncles, and my grandmother, who meant a great deal to me, had all produced children in their time. However, this distortion remained, and I was at a loss to decide what would or should a Mr Right in my life be like?

With the 60s came black is beautiful and hopes of some change for me. Black power meant Motown music, black singers in the record charts, and white people listening and enjoying Motown records. It was identifying with Angela Davis and her struggle, being sympathetic and sad about the Soladad brothers and again wanting to live in America, for very different reasons this time round.

It was only when Sandra, a black girl I'd known from school, came back into my life and we became good friends that my attention turned to black boys and men. At the time it all seemed wonderful. Positive images of black people were there in the culture at last. But the negative images of black women were still portrayed, including black men's images of black women.

This affected both Sandra and me. We thought the black boys we liked would now take an interest in us as young women whom they admired sexually. Instead, black men enjoyed this period by presenting themselves in a sexual way to white women, and we both found that it was black women, and not men, who used this time to address the politics of our blackness. It was not until many years later after reading numerous books on the black power movement, and in particular writing by black women, that the rejection of black women by black men became clear to me.

At the time, trying to come to terms with this as a black woman made me very unhappy. Apart from Sandra, there were other black women who became friends, girls in the local area. We identified with each other in a positive way. No longer did we want to straighten our hair. We were proud to wear our hair in the natural afro style. Before this time you always got called 'nappy head' unless you straightened your hair. We stopped experimenting with make-up that didn't suit us because it was not made for our colour skin. Despite this, black women had a struggle to be recognized and were still seen in a negative sexual light, whereas white women's sexuality was portrayed as beautiful.

For the first time I started to have a positive image of myself. Everything was exciting and new and I wanted to be part of the action. I wanted to shout to the world, *Here I am!* I was attracted by the women's movement but I felt frightened and sometimes angry, because the women advocating liberation were white. At that time they appeared to me as articulate, intelligent women who knew what they wanted. Although I felt at ease among them, I now believe they were patronizing. I could feel it but not identify it at the time. They were happy to have me along, but I always felt easily dismissed. My contributions appeared parochial in comparison with their discussions. It is only now that I realize how class and education played their part in this.

My image changed. I felt good and grew more creative. My feelings about what I wanted for myself developed. I decided that I would never marry or have children. I was reading lots of material about the women's movement and women's history. It all started to make sense. I decided that I would like to live and work abroad with women in third world countries. Their lives seemed so bad in relation to mine.

I admired the women involved in the women's movement. They were able to discuss openly the issues of sex and sexuality. Despite my new improved self-image I still had a different ideal of beautiful and sexually attractive womanhood. I didn't fit it. I used to think that white women acquired sex. Sexuality was something you bought if you had enough money. I wish now that I could have discussed these issues with my mother or grandmother, but I always found it impossible to start up a conversation on the subject.

The years from adolescence into womanhood steamed ahead for me. Although in some ways they were sad years, something did come out of them that gave me the determination not to give up on myself – to keep trying. I wanted to achieve something in life. But my involvement in the women's movement and the awareness that came out of it were short-lived. I seemed destined to go down a road that was typical of my circumstances and environment. Girls married young and had children. What was most common then was living in your parents' home with the extended family nearby.

Sandra and I used to go regularly to the local dance. It was there that I met James, who also was black and who was to become my husband for the better part of fifteen years. I liked James very much. He was quiet but appeared confident. What attracted me most was the concern he showed for me. He wasn't overpowering but he cared for *me* in particular. He made me feel great. He liked the way I dressed, the things we discussed, and most of all my personality. He took me to meet his friends and I was always over the moon when he told them I was his girlfriend. He always put his arms around me or held my hand when we were out. I thought this was wonderful. When I took him home my family liked him very much because he was reliable, had a steady job and was everything that a young man should be in their eyes.

We saw each other almost every night and would go out at weekends, sometimes getting back late. My mother didn't object to this because she knew I was safe with James. I was in love, or at least I thought I was. When we decided to go to bed together for the first time I didn't object or feel angry at his insistence. All I know is that I didn't see stars, hear music, or see rolling waves like in the films. After the first time it was easy to say yes and after a night out together we'd end up on the sofa in the front room at my house. I was a bit concerned because I did know you could get pregnant. What I didn't know was that some form of protection should have been used. James always assured me that it was OK and he seemed well satisfied, so I trusted him. But at the same time I felt guilty and wondered if anyone else in the house ever heard us, especially my mother. I used to worry in case someone walked in on us in the darkened room, so the experience was one of anxiety for me. I was also worried that if I didn't allow James to go all the way he might go off with someone else. The irony of all this was that I had only fully experienced sex maybe three times at the most when I became pregnant.

I didn't know at first what was happening to me, but by the third month and no period I realized what had happened. I didn't know what to do. How could I tell James? My first thoughts were that he would go mad. I felt so awful I couldn't face up to telling anyone. I wanted to run away, but where to? I even had thoughts of suicide. I had let everyone down and I felt sure my mother would kill me. I was in a state – no one to turn to, nowhere to go. I had heard about women having abortions but I didn't know where to go. The only place I had heard of was the Moral Welfare. I thought if I could find out where they were they might help me by sending me away to have the baby or else arrange an abortion for me. I remember walking around the town looking for the office, but I couldn't find it. My mind was a complete blank. I felt so guilty I didn't care what happened to me. These were the worst days of my life.

Eventually I went to the doctor's and told him I thought I might be pregnant – only to have it confirmed. Was there any way he could help me? He just looked at me, told me not to worry and gave me a note for the ante-natal clinic.

I had no choice now but to tell James. He went mad and called me everything. I told him that I had been to the doctor's but that he couldn't help me. James kept asking me to try and find someone who might be able to give me some tablets. By then I was a nervous wreck and was worried about having to face my mother and the rest of my family.

When we broke the news to my mother she called me all the stupid silly bitches going, reminding James that he should have been more careful. After a while things calmed down and my mother and auntie, along with James, arranged for the wedding.

I didn't have much to say about my own life now. Everything was said and done for me because I was the stupid one to go and get pregnant. We lived at my mother's house. We had our own bedroom, and made a contribution for our food, etc. The only time I went out during the next six months was to the ante-natal clinic, and even then my mother or aunt would come along with me. They asked the questions about me and the doctors would speak directly to them. I was never involved in the discussions. The doctor would examine me, ask how I felt and, before I had a chance to answer, would be saying, see you next week. I remember on one occasion the doctor asked me what size shoes I took. I thought they must be going to give me a pair of maternity shoes. Not until many years later did I come across the connection of small feet, small womb.

It wasn't until we left my mother's and went to live in a council flat that I got control of my life. I fulfilled my duties as mother and wife with vigour, doing housework all day. In the sitting-room we had a marly tile floor and I polished this every day. I felt it was so important to perform my duties very well. I was afraid that I would get pregnant again so I made sure I took the pill. I didn't know much about it, or the dosage or any kind of reaction that I might have. I was just glad that there was something that would stop me from getting pregnant. My sex life was just another household duty, the last thing to be performed at night, no pleasure for me at all. I just accepted this as how it was. As long as James was satisfied that was good enough for me. I never considered my own needs.

I had no social life. Only on rare occasions would we go to the cinema. I was an ardent reader of women's magazines. I didn't have any close friends on the housing estate and kept myself very isolated, just the occasional hello to my neighbours. I became friends with a woman called Diane at the school gate, and on the odd occasion we went shopping together after putting the children into school. Diane was very progressive in her outlook. She attended women's meetings, went on demonstrations, was involved in CND, etc. She would ask me along to these meetings but I never went. I thought I would be out of place because she knew lots of things and attended evening class. I admired her so much, but would not venture to think of changing my routine way of life. James would go out with his mates once or twice a week. I never went along. My only outing was to my mother's house on a Saturday after shopping or on a Sunday afternoon. James would drop me off there and collect me at 5.30 so I could get home and prepare the evening meal. There were times when I would have liked to stay longer at my mother's, but I knew James would not eat anywhere else except at home. I didn't resent this too much. In fact, I was grateful he had a good job. He gave all his money to me and I would budget to cover everything. I was very reliable and responsible where money was concerned. I never spent anything on myself unless I asked James first. I never felt the need to buy myself clothes or make-up. What I had was sufficient.

Slowly this began to change, and I realized that if I had a job and was earning my own money I could buy things for myself. I started looking for a job through the local papers. I was feeling bored with my routine way of life. The jobs that might have suited, and more importantly fitted in with my housework, were part-time typist vacancies. I came across an advert for a touch-typing course. Within twelve weeks you could be a proficient typist. The only snags were the £12 fee and the time – evening. I was very nervous telling James. I had worked it all out beforehand, informing him that my sister would come over from work and babysit, and his food would still be ready when he arrived home. I would be back in time to put the children to bed. Once I had the training I could get a part-time job. James agreed to let me go.

This move was the turning point in my life although I didn't realize it at first because my routine at home remained almost the same. I felt that if I was doing something for myself I must not inconvenience others. Obviously the guilt was still there within me.

I completed the course and tried to find a job. It wasn't easy. After numerous 'we'll let you knows' and direct 'nos' I realized for the first time that the main reason for these rejections was that I was black. I think it was the first time I'd experienced direct racism. I registered with every office agency and was unsuccessful with all of them. When I walked into an office the girls would look me up and down in surprise and inform me that they only offered office work. Reluctantly they'd take my details and say they'd get in touch with me, but they never did. I didn't give up. Week after week I'd do the rounds of the job agencies. They'd make up excuses – I was too late or they wanted someone with the relevant experience. How was I going to get the experience if they wouldn't give me a job?

I didn't tell James about their response. I felt he wouldn't believe me, or else he'd say, 'I told you so.' I was so unhappy. The only good thing that came about at that time was that James started working night shift. It was such a relief. By the time he got home in the morning I was up and busy. So it was only at the weekend that I had to endure my sexual relationship with him. I started to think about this, and occasionally I would say no or that I wasn't feeling well.

The excuses became more frequent. I got to hate having sex – there was no romance, no feeling for me. I don't think he ever told me once that he loved me. I thought for a while that he might be seeing someone else but I quickly did away with this idea. It was just me being nasty and horrible about him. His Saturday nights out continued every week. Occasionally he came back late but I would never question him. Apart from providing for my material needs he seemed indifferent. He never hugged me or kissed me apart from when we were in bed. I thought, I am reliable, responsible, look after him and his children, pay all the bills, and never ask for anything, so why would he want someone else? But my intuition was correct, though I didn't find out that he was having an affair until many years later.

I did another full-time office course. I arranged everything so that the house routine was not disturbed. James did not mind because life for him was still the same – meals always on the table at the correct time, clean house, clean clothes, even his shoes were polished. This time I was certain I would get a job. A part-time job did come up in a shipping office. The hours fitted in with my time, it was close by my mother's house so the school holidays would not present a problem. There were also plenty of shops nearby if I needed to shop during the lunch break. I was so anxious in case I failed once again.

When I arrived for the interview the personnel officer asked me what country I came from. I was shocked. Apparently the dole office clerk had informed him that I was a coloured woman, from Africa, she thought. I knew then I wasn't going to get the job. I was so hurt.

To my surprise a letter arrived the following day asking me to start on Monday. I worked hard at home, doing as much housework as I could. My first thought had been to tell James he could change the car because now I needed less housekeeping money. My mother on the other hand wanted to know why I wanted to go out to work but was satisfied when I explained how I'd worked out my routine and that neither James nor the children would be put out in any way.

I enjoyed working at the shipping office and picking up new skills, but I never went out with the girls from the office, even if it was Friday or someone's birthday. I knew I couldn't go out with them in the evenings even if I wanted to, so I never pursued this with James. I did start to buy myself clothes and make-up and get my hair done occasionally. Even so, I was very careful because I thought it was a luxury. James did notice the change in me and remarked on more than one occasion that my skirts were too short. When he was on nights and got up early in the day he would come and meet me from work.

The job lasted for just over a year, until the firm closed down and moved to a new development. They offered me a job with them but I had to turn this down as it was miles out of the city. It would have meant leaving early in the morning and getting home after James in the evening, so I was unemployed once again.

Soon I was back job hunting. This time I was experienced and had gained further skills but it still wasn't easy. I eventually got a job with a local welfare agency. Apart from typing and filing I was giving advice over the telephone directly to the public. I started to attend meetings in the evenings, taking the children with me. I attended courses on a variety of things. Even though I always arrived home before

9.30, James didn't like it. He would often start an argument with me – his food was cold when he arrived home, etc – despite the fact that a note would have been written letting him know the time I had left the house, where I was, and what time I would be home.

I never used to argue back, and said I would give up work if he liked so that I would not have to be out in the evenings. I wanted to keep the job but I also wanted to keep the peace at home. When we had an argument it was always me who said I was sorry, and I would try to make it up in bed with him even though I didn't want to. I was feeling frightened and thought I could not exist without James. Apart from making it all right with him sexually I would go out and buy him a new shirt or sweater to let him see I wanted him.

I kept my job and grew more involved. I attended day release courses and was always talking to James about the new friends I'd made. He wasn't interested, and when I started to invite people to the house he didn't like it at all. I knew our relationship was coming adrift. I was standing up for myself. James was now accusing me of going out with these men I was working with. It was the furthest thing from my mind. The men I came into contact with were pleasant and helpful towards me but I never found anyone in particular who was interested in me.

I started going away to weekend schools, always taking the children with me. Before and after my return James would cause such a fuss. During our arguments he would call me the most horrible names, like 'whore' and 'slut'. This upset me a great deal and made me start to question what I was doing. He would say that his friends were talking about me. What kind of man was he, allowing me to go away at weekends – I must be seeing another man? I wished at the time that I was. But on those weekends I was very guarded, and kept reminding myself that I mustn't relax, that I was there to learn and that any attractive remark or comment that was made to me by a man could not be true. When I was sitting close to someone I would find myself holding my body very stiff. I was frightened that if a man was to show any sign of sexual attraction towards me I just might not be able to control myself – against what I don't know.

I didn't realize then that I was a strong woman and could not easily be led in this way. But all the thoughts and reminders of what had taken place many years before at the time of my first sexual experience were still there, and I knew how vulnerable I could be. The thought of those years made me cringe. Although I wanted to be sexually attractive, I didn't feel it or believe that others would see me as such. I still felt awful when James called me names. For a long time I felt he might be right, so any sexual thoughts I had made me feel worse about myself.

My first sexual revelation came when I went away on a summer camp with the local residents' group. By this time I was doing my own thing as far as James was concerned, despite the arguments. That summer was very hot and we were camping. I was one of the camp leaders. There was also a priest from America and a young French student. After we'd got all the kids to bed we'd sit around the fire talking and drinking. It was wonderful. I think I fell in love with both the priest and the student. They often put their arms around me when we went out walking and my body felt very close to theirs. I found I was spending a lot more time on my appearance and often wondered if they noticed I was only wearing shorts and a thin T-shirt. At night I would often hope that they would come to my tent for something or other. A few years before I would have been worried about my sexual fantasies. Now I wasn't. Deep down I knew nothing would happen between us, but it was wonderful to experience that sexual feeling within me and to feel for the first time in my life that I was sexually attractive.

After that summer holiday I started to look after myself more. But the barriers I had put up around myself remained. I felt awkward when people, especially men, complimented me. I was working almost full-time and coming into contact with lots of people. They would say how good I was at my job and how nice I looked, but somehow I could not accept this. Looking back, the opportunity may have been there for me to have an affair but I dismissed any such thought immediately. My main aim was to do my job and do it more than well. As a black woman, people were always watching me and expecting me to fail. I passed a further course with high marks and began making decisions about my career.

I decided to attend a full-time course at an Oxford college. During the following months I was confused about what to do with the children. For the first time I wasn't worried about what would happen to James. I made my plans around childcare. Although my family was pleased, my mother just could not understand why I should want to go away and study. She was worried about James and about who would look after the children. Beneath all her doubts was the belief that going away to study was not a thing that a person like me should ever consider. I started to feel this also. But at the same time my mother wanted me to go, and soon she offered to look after the children. James was certain that with her care everything would go on as before. He was neither happy nor sad that I had been offered a place. He didn't stop me, nor did he encourage me. He knew that once I had made the final decision to go he had lost me.

I got the children into a local boarding school. My family was surprised and shocked. Little did they know that the decisive factor was the children settling into their new school. They went for a three-month trial period before I was due to go away. Everything worked out well. But the months leading up to my departure were a worrying time for me. Even though I had made my decision I believed that I was wrong to go on, that I was selfish, and above all that this was not for me.

The doubts and guilt remained with me the two years I was away despite everything working out all right as far as the children were concerned. Looking back now I do not know how I did it, or what spurred me on and kept up my morale. I was going to pack it all in on many occasions, because I thought I was taking too big a risk, trying to do something that wasn't meant for me, a black woman from my background. There I was, a black working-class woman sitting in a study room at an Oxford college. It didn't seem right. Many a time I would pinch myself, only to find out yes, it's real, and yes, it is me. I loved Oxford. It was everything I had read about and dreamt of. I was my own person there. People didn't see me through anyone else's eyes.

But I was also doubtful. I thought, this cannot last, something dreadful will happen and the whole experience will be gone in a flash. What also surprised and shocked me was that men in particular looked at me and passed positive comments. I couldn't take it and kept myself well guarded. I still did not trust them. My fear was that if I fancied someone in a sexual way the inevitable would happen. I had responsibilities back home and must not forget them. Every time someone passed a nice comment about me, or I fancied someone, I felt like giving myself ten lashes. I had come to Oxford to study, and must not allow myself any pleasures.

In my second year I lowered the barriers a little and did allow myself to become close to a man. I fell in love. I was frightened and never told him, but it was through him I became aware of my first real feeling of love, and we are still good friends today.

My best woman friend was Jean; I had made friends with her on my first day at college and she remained my strength throughout those years. Jean came from the north-east. She was married but had no children. We spent all of our time together and enjoyed each other's company. We had a lot in common – clothes, music, etc. It was great to have someone who really enjoyed me being around and could see my positive side. She helped me so much in many ways, knowing the difficulties I was under while at the college, and that I was under stress, although I never complained to her. Jean was so supportive, especially if I had had a bad week-end at home with James, which was often the case.

The children were no problem. They would come and spend weekends and half-terms down at the college. In the first year I was home almost every week-end. There used to be so many arguments between James and me. I was always glad to get back to college. It was like having a double identity. From Monday to Friday I would become the college student. From Friday evening to Sunday I would be the wife and mother. The transformation would take place at Birmingham on a Sunday evening where I would change trains. Jean would be waiting because she too would be returning from home. We used to laugh about the transformation as I got on to the Oxford train. I would stretch, take off the mother-wife cloak and put on my student cloak. I will always remember Jean for her kindness and the happiness she brought into my life those years at college. She often told me she also felt like giving up, but I would always encourage her.

It was a marvellous friendship and love between two women both going through changes for the better. Now when I look back at those years I can admit that I loved Jean but was afraid to tell her so. I think she knew. I will remember her not only for introducing me to Mocha coffee and Alliage perfume but for a kindness and support I never knew could exist between women.

When Oxford came to an end I was so unhappy, knowing I must go home even though I had the opportunity to continue on another course. I had a job waiting for me. Jean and I kept in touch for a time. She visited me occasionally but things were not the same. A different time, a different place. Another new cloak had been created for both of us. She divorced her husband, did another course, met the man who is now her husband, and had the child she longed for. I came back home and settled into my new life. I had changed into a different person. Although I separated from James about a year later, I continued to build on my new life with the children. I had the opportunity on a number of occasions to have relationships, but I was still afraid to get deeply involved with someone again. At least on my own I had the choice. I did have a couple of affairs and experienced sexual pleasure on my terms. If I had the chance again, of course, things would be different. We all say that.

I have only two regrets. The first is that I came to terms with my own self so late in life. The second is knowing that those first sexual experiences played a major part in my feelings and outlook about myself and life. When I was a girl I never in a million years dreamt that I would grow up to do the things I have done – making films, flying to Russia to meet the first space woman, developing my artistic qualities, doing a high-powered job, co-editing this book. I am an all-right person, and the damage and fear of my early life have been mended with time.

Longings to have the blinds up and the light on
Daisy McCauley

'*Now* can we have the blinds up with the light on?'

It was 1945. The war was over. I was five years old. A working-class child in Belfast, I longed for openness and freedom and for an end to the wailing and insistent sirens that signalled the rush to dark places and silence, where we would all be safe. I remember clearly asking the question.

When I reflect on these words it seems my life has been a journey – a journey that seeks for an end to silence. I wanted the blinds up and the light on so that I could see out and others could see in. The struggle has been ongoing, listening first to that part of me that says 'silence is safety' and that contrary aspect of myself that says 'silence is death'. Nowadays I listen to voices like that of Audre Lorde, speaking for millions of women, millions of lesbians like me:

> Our labor has become more important than our silence ... I have come to believe that what is most important to me must be spoken, made verbal and shared, even at the risk of having it bruised and misunderstood ... and it is never without fear; of visibility, of the harsh light of scrutiny and perhaps judgment, of pain, of death. But we have lived through all of those already, in silence, except death.

My need to write for this book comes from a desire to trace some of that life struggle, sharing where I've come from, and the place where I am now, for myself as much as for readers. Yet how ironic it is that I must write under a pen-name to protect others who feel that their lives would be ruined were they identified with me. I am reminded again and again of the compromises and constraints imposed on all of us lesbians by an oppressive society.

But let me start at the beginning and introduce you to my family. My father worked for thirty-five years for the same employer. When I meet new people it's important for me to say that – giving a message that whatever they think about the working class, *we* were respectable, honest, hard-working and loyal. We worked for the church, the orange order and the unionist party, and the local football teams. That was our life.

Our identity as a family revolved around my father – his job, his income, his standing in organizations that mattered. Still, it was my mother to whom he referred when decisions had to be made. Many a time I tried to get decisions out of him to which I knew my mother would not have agreed, but he always said, 'We'll see what your mammy says.' It was our mammy who managed the finances, who disciplined and defended us, who taught us to be independent and who resolved that all five of us would have a chance to be educated and 'cultured'. She made sure we all had piano lessons, and I went to elocution. If she thought complaints about her children justified, her wrath was formidable and her right arm like a heavyweight punch. We learned not to underestimate her, and because of her sense of justice and belief in our honesty, confidence was bred into us, and we knew we could trust in her ability to spot a liar. Only occasionally were we – and she – wrong.

Once I was considered old enough she went back to work, despite the protests of my father. He saw it as an affront to his role as breadwinner. But as in everything, she got her way. Work was a red-brick Victorian factory a short walk away. She started at 8 a.m. and finished at 6 p.m., and always came home at dinner time (also known as 'lunch'). When I visited her at work I found her in an enormous room of about 200 women, all in rows, all sewing handkerchiefs. There were several floors in the building, and a total workforce of about 600 women. When mother came home for her midday break she would snatch a doze on the settee. Often she'd tell us she had fallen asleep over her sewing machine.

My mother was considered very beautiful. Her hair was dark and her eyes a striking blue. She carried herself well and the only trace of self-worth I saw, was in her occasional boast that she was regarded as 'the straightest walker in the district'. Time and again my friends who met her remarked on what a good-looking woman she was. She remained so into old age.

Physically she was one of the strongest women I have ever met. She was capable of shifting large items of furniture, including our upright piano, did all her washing by hand, including four sets of football kit every Monday, and would stay up all night hemming, patching and ironing clothes to prepare for camp trips my brothers went on regularly (for some reason girls' organizations I belonged to never went to camp). Her health was excellent until in her mid fifties she suffered a mild stroke. She recovered almost totally and continued her life as before. She was seventy-nine the year she died.

My mother was born and lived all her life within a geographical area of about two square miles, although she travelled further abroad to visit her children once they'd moved away. Aged eleven when she started work, her life after marriage revolved around husband, family and political activities. She was taught that this was the normal expectation for all women.

I was my daddy's girl. After four boys my parents longed for a daughter, and I have always known how much I was wanted. My brothers said I was spoiled, but I didn't think so. I don't remember much before the age of five, though I'm told I was a happy child. I never had any sense of deprivation, mainly because my parents, and especially my mother, made invisible sacrifices to allow educational trips to France, or the piano lessons, or whatever was demanded as 'essential equipment' by the school. All five of us children had a chance to go to grammar school; three of us did. Of those three, it was my oldest brother who went on to university. Higher education was to come much later in my life, as it does for many women, if at all. My happiest memories are of spending every summer and many weekends in a rented thatched cottage — days of endless play and sunshine, jumping on and off hayricks and sliding down ditches, feeling free in my emerald green dungarees, so distinctive from my brothers' blue ones.

From my present perspective, accepting that we were working class and by no means well off, I see that we did have a lot of privileges unmatched by other families. Some of these extras resulted from our political connections, but nothing that was spoken of openly.

In Belfast, home was a terraced house with the front door on to the street — a nice, respectable street called an 'avenue' which was tree-lined. Those of us who lived in 'the avenue' were of the view that the other streets which ran parallel became increasingly inferior both in the house design and the quality of the area and the people who lived there. Our house had a parlour, kept for formal visitors and funerals, a kitchen (living room), a scullery (kitchen), two bedrooms and an attic stretching right across the house. There was no bathroom or inside lavatory. Our extended family occupied three houses in a row and another one across the street. I had a lot of contact with my aunts, uncles, cousins and grandparents, all of which reinforced the hard-working, 'respectable' ethos.

My brothers slept two in a bed in the attic and my parents had the front room. I had a room all to myself. I was highly ambivalent about that room. I loved its privacy and sanctuary but it emphasized my isolation, my 'difference', even before a consciousness about sexual identity emerged. It was a small room, containing a wardrobe with a long mirror, a dressing table and a tiny desk for me to do my homework. The bed seemed to fill the room, and the window looked out on our back yard. It seems now an austere little room. I slept in it until my late twenties and never had posters on the wall, nor do I remember pictures, or anything decorative that might have been described as colourful or bright. The lampshade was made of china, pale with delicate painted flowers. I was often terrified by a moth trapped inside it at night. Frantic to escape, it would tap ominously and insistently like the disembodied finger in stories my friends and I exchanged to frighten each other. I had nightmares and had a phase of bedwetting. A repeated nightmare was of me lying soundless and unmoving in a lion's den, so that I would be unseen both by the lions and by the people passing up and down a winding stair. Another was of running naked through empty streets or choking from a silent scream caused by an invisible terror. It was always my mother who appeared to comfort me. I often asked to sleep with my father – never my mother. They always obliged, and my mother would sleep in my bed. When I was thirteen and asked 'Daddy, can I sleep with you tonight?', his reply 'Not tonight' told me instinctively that I had slept with him for the last time. From then on there was no escape from my own sparse little room. It was there I comforted myself with my dolls, practising kisses on their cold mouths and struggling to work out how babies were made.

My class identity was a source of inferiority and shame from very early childhood. My parents associated with their 'betters' in the orange order and the unionist party, and worked for prospective councillors and MPs. The unionist MPs were inevitably from the Protestant ascendancy and were spoken of with awe and reverence. For my mother, places like hotels and restaurants were 'not for the likes of us', though my father was more defiant about his right to take up space. Even in later years when mother did consent to come into a restaurant, she was uncomfortable and embarrassed.

This sense of inferiority went deeper than class and extended to ethnic identity. When a male cousin married a woman from east London, a working-class cockney, my mother was paralysed in this woman's presence because she was 'English'. It was a strange contradiction. At school, in church, at home, we were imbued with a British rather than an Irish identity, prevented from learning about Irish history and culture, taught to revere the union jack and 'land of hope and glory'. At the same time, whatever way we turned, all the messages conveyed that we were inferior to the English.

Still, if we were inferior to the English, then we were certainly superior to Catholics. (*Roman* Catholic was the emphasis, symbolically underlining its sinister associations with the hated Pope.) I never met a Catholic until the year I was eighteen and working, and then generally relationships were characterized by mutual suspicion. I learned that you could recognize Catholics by their appearance, and indeed I could. In particular, their eyes placed closely together was a sign of their inherent untrustworthiness. (I later learned that Catholics were taught exactly the same about Protestants ...) Protestant children were warned never to go into a Catholic 'chapel', because they might not be seen again, and to avoid priests and nuns in the street, for fear of being kidnapped. When I was fourteen there was a highly sought-after book circulating which told horrific stories of sexual excess among priests and nuns, and of the existence of lime pits in convents into which the resultant unwanted babies were thrown. All Catholics were people to be avoided at any price. Then I encountered Maire, who shattered all my stereotypes about Catholics. She was my first real Catholic friend, when we worked together as clerks in the health service (regarded as the poor cousin of the civil service). She was sharp-witted, politicized and proud. I began to see that the 'look' which identified many working-class Catholics was one of dignity and defiance in the face of generations of oppression and blatant discrimination, and of being told this was not their country. Although I began to see, it was a long time before I understood. Maire's capacity to maintain a friendship while sustaining the challenge helped me along that road.

There have been a great many women who have influenced my life, and who have contributed in different ways to the shattering of silence and breaking down of barricades.

Lila lived a few doors away from us. We played ball and skipping, giggled a lot together and from the age of five were inseparable. We were simply, delightfully, very good friends. Now Elaine was different. She lived across the street, went to a different school from me, and somehow her family all seemed rather glamorous. Her looks and colouring were different from those of the rest of her family, with pale skin and red hair. We had a lot of fun, and at seven experimented sexually, examining and touching each other intimately. She came to our thatched cottage one summer, and the opportunity to sleep beside her was such a thrill. We planned to live together when we grew up. I still remember the disappointment when I realized that Elaine saw our planning as a game. After the sexual exploration with Elaine, I went on to discover boys. I was caught and punished in primary school for indulging in a mutual 'feel' with a boy during a lesson. The boy was caned.

With Julia my adoration was much more explicit. She had started grammar school a year before me. Tall and fair, talented as a singer and pianist, she lived in a nice house, and I thought her very grown-up indeed. Her father went to work in a suit and tie, and her mother baked caraway seed cake. I hated the taste, but suffered it in the name of love. Julia was involved in musical competitions and played the piano at social occasions at the church hall. Her best friend was Roberta. Right from the start I was on the sidelines, cycling round and round her street every day, hoping to catch sight of her. We seldom ever did anything together, and when I invited her to a special event with my parents she asked to bring Roberta too. Roberta came, and I felt keenly the disappointment of not having Julia to myself. I developed further the feelings of being an outsider, the recognition of 'difference', the feeling of being 'odd', isolated, secretive. My mother often accused me of never sharing anything with her, but how could I? My world shrank to my private thoughts and confusions, and *my* struggle to come to terms with the 'facts of life' seemed to hold no potential for dialogue with my friends at school, for the framework given to all of us was firmly a heterosexual one.

Once I went to grammar school I met Helen, and it was she who made the greatest impact on my young passions and my self-image, an impact that lasted for twelve years. We were in the same class. She was petite and attractive to boys. She too was talented musically. Her father had died when she was six years old. She and her younger sister had been brought up by their mother who struggled to maintain decent standards on a low income.

Helen told me recently that in her view it was the fact we were both 'different' that drew us to each other. We became good friends, and I fell silently and painfully in love. I gave her everything – my thoughts, my time, my loyalty, and most crucial of all, my capacity to think for myself. I listened to all she had to say, always approving and reassuring, and in my eyes she was incapable of error. But I had some measure of power and control too in that I was jealous of other friends, female and male. I demanded much of her time and was capable of producing sullen moods for lengthy periods. I never shared verbally my longing for intimacy – I'm not even sure that I allowed myself to think of physical contact beyond kissing her – and my internal struggles were not explicitly 'Who am I?' questions about identity. There was nothing nearly so articulate as that, much more about *I'm going through a phase – everyone goes through this phase*, and how I could deal with immediate feelings until the phase passed. It never occurred to me to question why, if I really believed this was a phase that everyone went through, it was not something that could be talked about openly. I guess I knew more than I was letting on, but chose to emphasize the 'common-sense' distortion about the 'phase' rather than to face the truth about myself at that time.

Not surprisingly I grasped every opportunity to be physically close to Helen, squeezed together in a car, or regularly sleeping together in her house or mine. When we slept together we would talk long into the night, having midnight feasts. My memory of this time is mainly of me listening to her intimacies and not having much to say for myself. Now I see that I resented Helen for this. She left school at fifteen, as many working-class kids did. Partly she was disenchanted and humiliated by the system, and partly her mother needed the extra income. I decided to leave too, and began to look for a job in every hardware shop, baker's and grocery store on our road. One of the shopkeepers told my mother, who promptly put an end to any ideas about leaving school, so I stayed and did O levels.

It was during that first summer when Helen started work that our relationship touched a crisis. Her mother and sister had gone on holiday and I moved into her house for two weeks. She went to work every day and I waited for her to come home. I don't remember how I spent the long hours, but there was enough time for my imagination to burn. I had fantasies about our bodies being very close and what it would be like if we kissed and held each other. Day after day these thoughts were all I could allow into my head, until I lost all judgment and perspective. I was incapable of thinking beyond the actions to their consequences. I began to believe that she wanted what I wanted. And I kissed her. Suddenly, clumsily, passionately, in bed. We never spoke of it again, not even to this day, though we have talked openly about our different sexual choices. Her shock and horror stunned us both into rigid silence, staring disbelieving into the dark night, with me wishing I was dead.

Our friendship continued as before, with no apparent difference. Then Helen became involved in a fundamentalist, evangelical Christian group – and so did I. Such churches have been popular in industrial, working-class areas, and offer purpose and salvation in the next life as well as in this. The way services are conducted is lively and vital. Commitment and sacrifice are demanded from – and wholeheartedly given by – the members. Such churches give power and punch to religion, and make it relevant to working-class cultures in a way that many traditional churches cannot. At the same time, they tend to be ultra-conservative, forbidding sex before marriage, disapproving of divorce, shunning alcohol and tobacco, and demanding withdrawal from 'the world'. Men are seen to be the god-ordained masters of women, and the concept of women's liberation is a travesty of the divine economy. To be gay or lesbian is anathema, and is regarded as the ultimate perversion.

For the next fourteen years I threw myself into every aspect of the sect. The most important consequence was that I did not have my first fulfilled relationship with another woman until I was thirty. I suppose at some level my entry into religion was an attempt to avoid the reality of my sexuality, but I was not and never have been consumed with guilt about my loving women. The social messages were confusing but remorse and guilt were not significant features of my experience. I am sure that by far the stronger motivation was the desire not to be parted from Helen and the urge to continue a relationship with her, however vicarious.

There were many satisfactions in being a member of the church. Although women were barred from positions of office or power, they were encouraged to pray publicly and to preach. I became their star 'lady' preacher, and did this regularly once a month for several years. I was given respect and status, and fostered a sense of self-worth and identity. Within the restricted framework I experienced a measure of empowerment, and of development of skill and ability. I am sure there are many women with a similar experience, while many of us outside it wonder incredulously how they can tolerate such oppressive situations. Although for me there was this sense of empowerment, it did not in itself hold any potential for my journey out of darkness. My window-blinds stayed firmly shut.

Helen was not particularly impressed, and preferred to see a man in a pulpit. It was somehow more 'natural' she said, though her role as a musician was as important to her as mine was to me. The years passed, the friendship continued and we each became more deeply involved in church activities. When Helen was twenty she married a preacher and moved away. My tie to her was no less secure, the pain was no less real, but by this time I had become remarkably self-contained, and expected nothing from relationships with women beyond 'lasting friendship'. Those who did recognize my moroseness interpreted it as disappointment at my not yet having 'found a man' of my own. They reassured me 'my turn would come'. During the period in which I knew Helen I was attracted to a number of women, mostly where I worked. Some of these attractions grew out of friendship, but I experienced periods of being 'weak at the knees' about women I hardly knew. I never uttered a word about these feelings to anyone, nor did I explore the implications too deeply with myself. There were men too that I met and liked. These relationships were superficial and short, and usually with men in the church who admired my 'spirituality'. I think I persuaded them that I was a 'creature apart'!

I became more and more restless in the church. I would have liked to progress, but there was no future for me there, and I became increasingly aware of and resentful of its oppression of women. I had been in a clerical job for nine years, and knew I was capable of something more. So when a job in social work came up, I went for it. There were fifty applicants, and what a boost it was to be the one offered the job. Now I know that my mother had had a word in the ear of a city councillor.

For eighteen months I learned about social work and gained enough experience to be accepted on a training course. Then I was on my way to England to live and study away from home for the first time in my twenty-nine years. There I found Mary, and finally, myself.

Like me, Mary was an Irish Protestant. We were students on the same course. For the next two years we studied together, played together, spent all our time together, talked endlessly about social issues, and six weeks before our course was due to end, made love together. It took a long time to get to that bedroom scene, because certain events associated with my attempts to hold on to the church connection intervened, the most significant of which was my engagement and impending marriage to Richard. He was from a rival Christian sect, preoccupied by his own sense of sin and guilt, yet sensitive and informed and generous. Our courtship was conducted between Belfast and Liverpool, both passionate and ambivalent, until finally six weeks before the wedding I realized I couldn't go through with it. All this now seems rather irrelevant, but it is with enduring vividness that I remember the chaos I created by calling the whole thing off, and my mother's response. She was wonderful. Instead of hostility to this totally unexpected news, she accepted my decision and gave her full support to it. Maybe she knew more than I did?

My decision wasn't because I had realized I was a lesbian, for although I was now thirty, I still had not arrived at that obvious conclusion. I reasoned that we 'were not right for each other' as individuals. Still, it was a watershed because it released me from the social pressure to marry, and Mary and I shared our bodies and our love. I knew then that I had come home. She asked, 'Does this mean we're lesbians?' I said I didn't think so, but deep down I knew. There was no sense of unnaturalness, not a hint of guilt, no wondering what it all meant. No questions needed to be asked, no answers needed to be given. Sounds like the end of the journey, does it not? But no, as it turned out it was simply like changing trains towards a still uncertain destination.

Mary and I had six weeks of dizzy romance before we both returned to Ireland to the serious business as social workers in our war. We lived 100 miles apart, and saw each other every second weekend in the house Mary shared with her father. Although he knew we slept together, we all three pretended it was as 'good friends'. Mary never did accept a lesbian identity, and she married eventually. As for me, I was delighted with this lesbian love that was at last fulfilled. We lived it rather than talked about it, and entered wordlessly into a pretence that our relationship was a close friendship. Holidays were the best times because then *everything* was unreal and so provided a measure of consistency between us and the rest of the world. Mary was full of laughter and fun, she was warm and welcoming to everyone she met. We wanted to be together and started making plans. At last she got a job in Scotland, and I determined that I would find one too (why am I always following women?). I was living alone with my mother then, and I recall with shame how I announced to her that Mary was going to Scotland. Mum was in hospital recovering from a hysterectomy when I told her. 'You'll be going too, won't you?' she said. I was dumbstruck. How could she know what was in my mind?

When Mary left for Scotland her father went too. Mary didn't seem to make any effort to dissuade him so our plans for living together were dashed. At that point, neither of us regarded our relationship as legitimate enough to have any right to expect fulfilment without inconvenience. Unhappy but fully accepting the situation, I arrived and stayed with Mary and her father for three fraught and frustrating months. Finally I found a place of my own nearby, a lovely old flat, the very first home I had ever owned. I had already found a job before coming, in a voluntary social work agency. Our secret life continued as before, more or less.

Because of my job I was forced for the first time in my life to confront the realities of class difference at every turn. The agency's origins were born of *noblesse oblige* and its dominant culture was genteel middle-class professionalism. For the life of me I couldn't understand why they appointed me, since the only other working-class staff were the secretaries (and I knew this time there was no city councillor involved ...). They had appointed Susan, whose origins were in lower middle-class Belfast, at the same time as me. She had been to university and her father was a teacher, so she seemed more able to cope with it all. The culture, the values, the language of these refined women were quite foreign to me. I literally could not understand what people were saying to me, even though I recognized individual words. The way sentences were constructed seemed to me to be so obscure and circuitous that it made no sense to a woman accustomed as I was to direct and unambiguous speech. I was disempowered and angry, and for the next four years fought my way through that job, challenging and being challenged at every point. In the early days I found sanity from three main sources – from the single parents who were my 'clients', from Mary, and from Susan, who was strong, easy-going, soft and humorous. She too was to become my lover.

Susan is also Irish. I should warn now that you are to read that statement once again before my story ends! Her living arrangements were breaking down at the time I was moving out of Mary's house into my own flat, so she moved in with me. Over the next year my relationship with Mary continued, with her coming to sleep with me regularly. Nothing was said to Susan, and she apparently did not put two and two together. It is amazing how perceptive people often do not see what is under their noses, yet when they are told realize they have 'known' all along. My friendship with Susan grew and matured over the next year, and then, when she was about to move into a flat of her own, we quietly, gently, unremarkably became lovers. The friendship that had developed among the three of us then became a triangle.

Oh, what a tangled web! I told Susan about Mary, and we argued the pros and cons of being honest with her. We owed it to her as a friend, and what if she ever found out? But wouldn't our friendship be damaged? Could we risk wrecking something so good? How hurt she would be. Surely it would be better to leave things as they were? And that's what we decided to do. Having agreed to deceive Mary, Susan and I entered into an unspoken, collusive pact not to discuss the matter again. We pretended the deceit wasn't happening. For a while Mary continued to spend nights with me, sometimes unexpectedly letting herself in. Hearing the key grate in the lock, Susan would scramble out of my bed (the only double bed) with a now familiar sense of panic. I could not maintain the pretence of making love with Mary. Gradually that part of our relationship withered away, but again there were no words to record the change. It was as though Mary had joined in the deceit, avoiding asking painful questions for fear of ruining our friendship.

The three of us became inseparable. We were together at every opportunity. We went on holiday, ate, played, visited together. Friends later said they found it impossible to offer an invitation to one without offering it to the other two, which must have made entertaining us a real drag. As time went on it became easier for me to carry the unease and guilt, and eventually I forgot that I was living a dishonest life. Perhaps the difficulties were lessened because most of my life before then had been like a tightly closed book anyway, so this wasn't really so different.

What can I say about all this? The way Susan and I behaved was cowardly and mean, and in the end caused enormous damage to all three of us. There are no excuses for it. We knew from the start that we were wrong. The lies we created are no different from and no more justifiable than those found in many relationships. Are there any elements that are different? We existed outside the accepted, unquestioned structures that tell us what we are meant to believe about sex and sexuality. Lesbian relationships are illicit, therefore any question of morality in conducting them is spurious. They must be kept well away from the light of day – not to be given legitimacy by any discussion of them. In any case, sex is a private matter and not part of every-day conversation. These were the structures that cheated us of opportunities to open our lives to each other and to other lesbians, that robbed us of their company and self-affirmation, even of knowledge of their existence. It was in a context of isolation, of unrecognition, of silence, that our actions took shape. Saddest of all now is the thought that each one of us thought so little of ourselves and each other that we were prepared to settle for a farce.

We lived in this way for more than two years. I found the triangle more and more intolerable. It became so suffocating I wanted to scream, and often did. Each of us tried to widen our independent social contacts, yet constantly found ourselves drifting into the old pattern. After all, it was familiar and appeared to offer security. The volcano erupted when I fell for Maureen. Of course I was looking for a way out, but I am certain that a good part of my attraction to her was due to her insistence on honesty in personal relationships. It was then 1978, and through many ups and downs I have loved her ever since. Two years before, she had come to the same agency where Susan and I worked, and we all liked each other instantly. Maureen was middle class like the other staff, but her ability to communicate with people from all walks of life made her popular with most people. Her warmth, her directness brought new vitality and freshness to a staid and traditional office.

Maureen is a Scot with lots of physical energy and versatility, and excels at any sport she has tried, especially swimming. Outgoing and extrovert, she is at the same time introspective, reflective and interested in mysticism. When I got to know her she was deeply into the philosophy of Hinduism and Buddhism. These very different elements in her personality make her endlessly interesting and challenging, and for the two years we'd worked together I'd admired her and found conversations with her always food for thought. It had never occurred to me she might be a lesbian, so convinced was I that there weren't many around. I do remember though, at one point, experiencing a fortnight of intense attraction for her which I found disconcerting. Then it was gone, at least temporarily.

It was after a row we'd had at work and a drink at a pub to sort it out that she told me she was 'bisexual' and I told her that Susan and I had 'more than a friendship'. Very soon, when the implications of that exchange of information sank in, we were in each other's arms. I knew I had to tell her all, for otherwise the intrigue would deepen. I was convinced she would immediately reject me. On the contrary, her confidence in my basic integrity helped me to begin to unravel the mess.

Susan had to be told about Maureen, and Mary had to be told about both Susan and Maureen. The months that followed were nothing less than a nightmare. Mary sank into a deep depression and blamed Maureen for everything. Nevertheless, she had started a battle for survival which she has won, and has rebuilt her life. Susan was shattered but kept a tight rein on her feelings, and speedily found a man to marry. Her lifelong fear of depression and loss of emotional control seemed to carry her through the crisis.

For Maureen and me, life was far more complicated than each of us finding a new lover. Thoughts of a 'happy ever after' scenario were quite unrealistic. I had just started a research job, and Maureen was on her way to a job in India for four years. Although she had known about her lesbian identity from an early age, she was now considering whether life might be easier as a heterosexual. From March 1978, when we first 'discovered' each other, until October 1979 when her visa for India came through, we struggled with complex and contradictory forces. There was the constant mending, restoring and re-forming of friendships we were striving for with Mary and Susan, and which we never achieved. With Susan the hurt and damage were too deep for any element of trust to grow, and with Mary the need to blame someone was too strong to be overcome. They formed an alliance with each other which cast them both as victims and united them against Maureen in particular.

Alongside all this, Maureen and I were working to cope with a parting that we knew to be inevitable, but with no idea when it would be. Maureen was confused over whether she wanted to love women but knew she loved me. She was anxious about facing a long, lonely time in a new and strange culture. For my part, I was angry and bewildered that she could leave someone she loved, yet I could also accept and dimly understand that she needed to go. I was in a new job and living alone for the first time in my life. There was no security for either of us, and any long-term commitment was out of the question in these circumstances.

Then she was gone. It was months before I recognized that I had sunk into a state of depression. I got on with life; met new and subsequently dear friends through my job at the university; went through the motions of living. The most important link with life was the routine of walking and feeding my dog. Every day, regularly, he insisted on being attended to, and I responded. Those solitary walks on the beach, those familiar but safely distant faces of other dog-walkers, little Sandy's trusting and unjudging companionship, all spoke of security and tomorrow.

While Maureen was away, two other women held deep significance for me, and I am pleased that I have their friendship still. The first was Sinead, whose Irishness is important because of her sense of herself as an *Irish* woman, which challenges me to rethink my ethnicity and nationality, and has helped me to recognize how this had been fragmented and distorted by my Ulster Protestant culture. A more immediate impact was her opening up for me a new feminist perspective on the world which was both exciting and discomforting, touching in me deep whispers long familiar yet unknown. Until then I had known little about feminism and the insights it might hold for me. My sense of injustice was individualized, with very little sense of the links with other women's experience. Sinead opened the way for that connection to be made. She is vivacious and volatile, demanding, generous and passionate. When I met her, I had not moved on from Maureen. That is why much of the short period with Sinead was unhappy and frustrating.

Through Sinead I was introduced to the women's movement, to books, ideas, films, to women who were making sense of their experiences of gender, sexuality, class, race, in a way that began to transform my instinctive feminism into a coherent and political whole. Most of all, these were women who were determined to end the silence, to have the blinds up, to see and be seen. With their help, and with their tugging at the sash, not always gently, my blinds began to give way. The transformation for me is not complete. I don't anticipate that it ever will be, because the struggle has to be engaged in daily, and because new experiences add new insights and dimensions to my understandings. But I am grateful to Sinead for the push she gave me into a place where eventually I felt I belonged.

The friendship with Sinead survived and matured, a lasting tribute to the potential for women to love each other in a world which treats us, and holds a danger in our treating each other, as sexual objects. And strange as it may seem, thousands of miles away in India, through the love of another woman, Maureen too was finding her own feminist perspective, and learning to value herself as a lesbian. For both of us, a foundation was being laid which would give our eventual decision to live together a reasonable chance of survival.

When Virginia burst upon me she was twenty, a second year undergraduate. Tall and lovely, she looked sometimes so elegant and sometimes so gauche, but always vital and endearing. Virginia was 'out'. Her favourite badge said 'Every woman is a lesbian'. She was unmistakable because she loved to dress up. Her best outfits were her Nell Gwynne (the basket always had a packet of fags and matches instead of oranges), and her French prostitute – including the beret.

Occasionally she might turn up in long johns and a vest, and wearing an enormous white garden-party hat. Always with all of these outfits went the Doc Marten boots. The overall effect was a stunning message that said 'I don't give a fuck what this world thinks, and will do as I like.' Virginia was non-monogamous, which I agreed with in theory but found hard in practice (mainly because it was *her* non-monogamy and not mine). She brought gaiety back to my life. I was beginning to be my own person and now had a confidence that I would stay in one piece, whatever happened. Virginia enriched (and still enriches) my life enormously, with her determination to defy falsehood and pretence, and her love of life and creativity. We had a short six months together, and now have a lifetime of friendship.

Maureen's job in India ended in 1982. After those agonizing years apart she at last decided she wanted to be with me. I joined her for her last four months in India and we began the job of getting to know each other again, but this time from a position of greater personal strength and clarity. Our relationship will always be volatile and intense, both in passion and depression, but we're each sure of our identity and the road we want to travel together. In saying this I do not want to underplay the lasting damage to self-confidence that is inflicted by a society bent on control, by distortion of what we know and understand. As lesbians we are confronted daily with the need to spend our energy on 'holding on to ourselves' in situations that threaten to crush our sense of being. We now know we are not alone.

As for me, the work on the politics of identity – gender, sexuality, ethnicity, nationality, class, culture, and now increasingly, aging – goes on. The blinds continue to shorten. I'd like to say that one day they suddenly shot up with a dramatic crash and the sunlight streamed into my sparse little bedroom. That could complete the imagery in a piece like this. But no, I cannot report such an event. The work is hard and, I suspect, will occupy me for my lifetime.

It is only recently, for example, after nearly forty years, that I have taken back the last vestiges of the control I had surrendered to Helen. Gradually I began to recognize the oppressiveness of the relationship. When she informed me that Maureen and I would not be permitted to stay overnight (the dreaded bedroom scenario) in her house if we visited Ireland, I knew it was time to finish the friendship. I was able to do this not with pain or even regret but with relief and a surge of strength, and with resolve not to turn back.

Audre Lorde's voice has been ringing in my ears as I have written these final pages, reminding me again of the risks of sharing – of having what is important bruised, misunderstood and judged. I can have no control over reactions to what I have written. But I am glad the silence is broken.

No longer a victim
Anji Watson

I grew up in a household where sex and sexuality were not talked about. There were no avenues open for discussion, questions or childish curiosity. The subject of sex was simply taboo. My mother was religious, fanatical about us kids being in church every Sunday. She taught us to be good for God because he was everywhere and knew everything. The big emphasis was on confession – if we sinned we must confess to the priest. With the stain of sin on our souls we could not go to mass, no, that would have been very bad, that was the way with Catholicism. My father was indifferent to all this, removed from what was happening around him. He was Welsh and had gone to work for a time in Holland where he had met my mother. They got married and she came back with him to live in England.

I went through the ceremonies of holy communion and being confirmed; dressed all in white, so deeply representative of virginity. I liked the attention and the dressing-up but the idea of God freaked me out. The thought of him being everywhere made me self-conscious about masturbating. Masturbation, which I began when I was about eight, was my guilty secret. In bed, under the covers I explored my body and worried about God watching me, judging me. I came to see this habit of mine as naughty, sinful and shameful.

The year I was eleven I tried to penetrate myself with a bangle. I'd fashioned it into an oblong shape especially for the purpose. Despite continued efforts I had to give up trying because I'd made my vagina so sore. There was the familiar guilt afterwards and a whole lot of confusion as to why I was trying to do this to myself. Now, I can understand that my feelings about masturbation were mixed up with feelings about being sexually abused.

It was my brother who abused me. He was sixteen the year I was seven and that was when it began. It happened over a period of eighteen months. Then he left home and the opportunity was no longer there. I've written poetry and filled diaries with my anger. What he did robbed me of my childhood innocence and there are times when I feel full of grief for that small girl so unprotected and vulnerable. So much of what happened has gone from my mind but there is one particular incident that I have not been able to forget. He used to take me to play with him; that's what he used to say to me and my mother, and those words have an odd, menacing ring as I put them down on paper. This one time he had a few friends along to play too. They took me to a secluded area and told me they wanted me to take my pants off. I sensed something was very wrong and in panic ran away, afraid and very confused.

In later years there were other situations where the same sort of fear and confusion took hold of me, though outwardly I pretended to be coping quite well. At primary school some of the boys got a group of us girls to meet them in a far corner of the playground. They said they'd show us their dicks if we, in turn, showed them our private parts. Seeing how reluctant I was one boy tried to manipulate me by saying he'd not be my boyfriend any more if I didn't show them my cunt. I refused but was very upset. I hadn't known he was my boyfriend, what did he mean?

Another time, another public toilet. Teenagers now, my girlfriends act competitively towards each other, the boys are lecherous and leering. I'm the last one to show myself and I only do it because I feel unable to say no. One of the boys tells me, after whispering it to everyone else first, that I'm not the slag I make myself out to be. Hurt, I wonder what he means by this remark. He was right though. I had to portray myself as being 'up-front' and open about sex, but it was all bravado. I could never let on that really I was scared and confused; I always had to be seen as being in control. I certainly wasn't as easy-going about my sexuality as I would have others believe.

It was during my teen years that I felt most inadequate. It was a difficult period. The other girls had rounded breasts and full figures, while my body was small and not defined at all.

How to describe my experience then? It was like a rollercoaster that was out of control. Two important factors greatly influenced my life during those years. The first was getting into trouble with the police; the second was more sexual abuse.

We moved from Nottingham to a small village when I was twelve. At school my accent was noticeably different and the other kids poked fun. I was also shy and passive. I hated being the new girl at school. Soon, they weren't just calling me names but waiting for me after school. There'd be a whole crowd of them trying to goad me into starting a fight. Aware of what would happen if I did, I ignored them as best I could. Everywhere I went in that village there was someone from school making threats or passing on a message that so-and-so was out to get me. It got worse and worse. I was intimidated and constantly anxious. Then, suddenly, there was Alex. She wasn't popular either. Alex came from a large family and was considered scruffy. I remember her as solid and brave. She used to get bullied too. We were together through months of this sort of treatment.

My mother worked at the school as a cleaner. I'd told her several times what had been going on but she never took me seriously until the day I told her I wanted to die. Nasty letters had been arriving through the post. That was the last straw. I couldn't eat or sleep nor could I concentrate on anything. My mother went to see the headmistress even though I pleaded with her not to. I was called in and asked to tell my story then the bully girls were sent for. Left alone in the headmistress's office my mother unexpectedly pulled me on to her lap. I was embarrassed. She never hugged or cuddled me at home and it felt inappropriate to be doing it there and then. It was more like a fight than a cuddle. I struggled to get down. Why was my mother going on like this? My tormentors were reprimanded that day and the bullying stopped. I was very relieved.

I saw less and less of Alex after that. Now I had Penny as my close friend. Penny had big breasts and I was fascinated by them and by her. I was intrigued and infatuated by her, partly because she seemed so grown up. I wanted to be like her.

Penny was into sexual games played out with boys and I was there to be partnered with the mate of the boy she'd picked. The pattern became predictable – kiss, fondle, finger-fuck. I never went further than the fondling and was completely freaked out if a boy asked me to wank him. I did have sexual feelings towards girls but had not yet developed desire for boys. Penny seemed to think that boys was what it was all about, so I thought I should think that way too. My friendship with Penny worked like this — she would fix us up with boys, and in exchange I'd take her shoplifting with me.

Our friendship ended when we got caught running off with a T-shirt from C&A. We were taken to the local police station where we each made a statement, then had to wait around for hours before our parents came to collect us. In court, we were given unconditional sentences. It was all over very quickly. The worst thing for me was having to endure my mother acting like a martyr at the police station. She cried and went on and on. Once home, my father gave me a good hiding.

I soon found a new lot of friends and some of the girls who had bullied me were in this new group. This was the time of the skinhead era and we were keen to dress the part with an intense sort of vengeance. Crombie coats, staypress trousers, Ben Shu shirts and loafers or brogues — this was our uniform. To have status in the group you had to have fights. We were quite intimidating. I soon became a bully. I never had a lot of fights but I learned to use my mouth instead of my fists. I managed to get those bully girls ostracized from the group, and oh boy, was revenge ever so sweet? But I didn't let it stop there. I always took risks. I wanted to be daring and popular among my peers. I was angry and took it out on anyone who got in my way. I had no respect for authority, other people or myself. I was headed for trouble and I got it too.

It was Halloween night. A whole gang of us decided to run riot through the village. We rampaged through the streets, pounding on people's front doors, throwing bangers through letter boxes, and while we called it fun, we must have been a nuisance to everyone else.

We drifted towards the school grounds. Some of the boys managed to break in while the rest of us broke aerials of cars parked nearby, or let the air out of numerous tyres. Back on the streets we picked on a girl who was walking by. The police were called and there was a mad chase with many of us hiding from the police in the graveyard. One boy was caught, taken to the police station and left in an interview room. He escaped through a small window but was caught again later on. He told them all they wanted to know.

The next day at school we were all interrogated by the head teachers and the police. I was scared and excited. I told them everything they wanted to know and they commended me for my honesty. Only two of us went to court, me and Laura. We were charged with causing grievous bodily harm to the unsuspecting girl who'd got in our way. At court, we sat on a wooden bench in front of the magistrates. I was blasé about the whole thing and at times wanted to burst out laughing. All those official-looking people bustling about in black cloaks with very serious faces. We two sniggered and giggled whenever possible. There were people frowning at us in all directions during the proceedings. We got a telling off and a fine for our misdemeanours. My father was so angry about me laughing in court he thumped me several times around the head. He often hit me around the head; sometimes he'd hit me so hard my head would bounce off the wall. The next week in a school corridor I overheard one teacher comment to another that I was more disturbed than Celia Thomas. Celia lived on a council estate and, though she was considered a bit slow by the teachers, I knew how well she spoke with her fists. I thought she was dead hard so considered the comparison a compliment.

We had to move again because of my father's job. This time it was a large town in the Midlands. I didn't want to go; Laura's family had said I could live with them but my parents had said no, I was too young. I felt I was being wrenched away from everything that was important in my life.

My bad reputation worked to gather girls around me at the new single-sex school. Five of us truanted one day, spending the time at Dee's place while her mother was at work. We got to messing about with the phone and, when it was decided to make bomb threat calls to schools in the area, I was persuaded to make the calls. Practising an Irish accent and taking advantage of a lot of IRA activity in England around that time I phoned three schools, including my own. We were surprised and alarmed when, later that day, two policemen came knocking on the door. It seems the police and school staff had collected names of children not in school that day and the police were systematically calling at each home to check the legitimacy of excuses given for absence. Dee spilled the beans quickly and wailed like a baby. The rest of us slipped away, over the back fence, but we'd all heard Dee blabbing and knew what was going to happen. I don't remember much about being arrested.

This time the court scene was high drama. Dee pleaded not guilty and her mother had a lot to say about who was really behind all this. The rest of us pleaded guilty and I was soon pushed forward as the ringleader. Dee's solicitor gave me a hard time, Dee fainted and I had an anxiety attack. We were both carried out of court. All five of us were fined and placed on probation. After the case was over my mother made arrangements for me to be referred to a psychiatrist who promptly prescribed Valium. I was fifteen. Even though I saw the psychiatrist for some months she never did uncover the fact that for the previous two years I had been sexually abused and beaten regularly, by my father.

My father was quite subtle in the way he manipulated me and there were so many times that I felt anger, hatred and shame. He found different ways of abusing me and the following example tells the story of just one incident.

We were alone in the house. Mum was working, she was always working. I had a cold. He told me to get the jar of Vick so he could rub my chest.

Unsure of what he intends to do, I stumble around the room but I dare not disobey him. I hand over the jar and he takes it and smiles at me. I can feel myself cringing, and drop my eyes to the floor.

'Lift up your jumper.'

I stare at him blankly.

'Come on silly, I'm only going to rub your chest.'

I lift up my jumper.

'Now your bra.'

I can't move, I feel rooted to the spot.

'Come on darling, it's only your dad, you can trust me.'

I do as I'm told. I hate it. He rubs my chest and fondles my breasts. My skin is burning; my breasts feel like they might explode. I'm going to burst into flame any minute now. I hate it. I hate it.

There is no memory loss around the abuse I suffered from my father. Many times I have wished for blissful oblivion.

I coped by being two different people. One Anji was out on a stage, acting up, kicking over the traces. The other Anji was introverted, held down, packed in tight. At home I was quiet and withdrawn but I had rebellious outbursts, mostly with my mother. I steered clear of my father. His violence was unpredictable and scary, but fortunately he wasn't around a lot. On the streets I was loud and cheeky. I never cried in front of anyone, and whenever I saw or noted anything upsetting I laughed to hide my real feelings. There were times when I did cry, alone. It was a very private act. I know now that many women enduring sexual abuse withdraw to some distant, unapproachable place inside. Only in the last few years have I been able to learn how to be myself. I'm almost ready to tell my mother what my brother did to me, but when, if ever, will I be able to tell her about my father? I don't know. I'm getting stronger but I no longer overestimate that strength, the way I used to as a child.

My father's work took him away from home for nine months the year I was sixteen. I made some changes while he was gone. First I stopped taking the Valium and then I got a job, at Woolworth's. Much to everyone's surprise, I got on well there and began training as a supervisor. Things went well until the day I blew it and got caught pinching a pair of socks. Of course I was sacked on the spot. The humiliation was unbearable. Sitting in a small room at the police station I bit off every single one of my fingernails. I loathed myself completely. My mother was playing the martyr again. Where had she gone wrong, she asked, shoulders shrugging, hands upturned, the very picture of suffering and despair? I know she did have cause for concern. She had such a need to stay in control of events and I must have seemed uncontrollable at that time.

My probation officer kept me from being taken into care. His liberal approach annoyed my mother. He was too soft, she complained. They had one row after another and he had to stop coming to the house, she was so disagreeable. My relationship with my mother had become full of bitterness and resignation. She knew nothing about me; knew nothing about the things I had coped with. She hadn't protected or saved me from my brother or my father. I knew I didn't blame her for that, but accepting the overwhelming reality was sad and inescapable.

I was always pushing her.

I wanted her to be different.

Why couldn't she see what was happening to us?

She had three children to look after and an alcoholic husband who beat her. He was also unfaithful to her. She was angry about his love affairs and would not let him get away with deceiving her. She fought him yet she accepted him too. I ask myself now, if there were things she chose not to know? My problem was that I knew too much, knew things she didn't, couldn't, wouldn't, know. The daily grind of poorly paid work tired her out and robbed her of health and energy to do other things. She wanted us kids to stay in line so she could just get on with each day as it came. No wonder our relationship was appalling. What chance did we have?

I did try to win her approval. It was one of my jobs to vacuum and dust while she went shopping on Saturdays. One week I did a brilliant job and Mum was very pleased. But whenever I cleaned up after that she would always compare it to that earlier time and my latest efforts never quite measured up. She used to hit me and yell that I'd let everyone down – her, my father, my sisters, even myself. Ours was a love-hate relationship for a very long time. But, chastened by my latest destructive episode, I did hold on to some hope about the future. I hadn't been carted off to some institution for wayward girls, so that was something to be grateful for. Eventually I found another job. It was then that I left home. I was seventeen. Mum and I never spoke for a long time.

Soon after leaving home I was attacked by a man I met in a pub. He wasn't local, we weren't exactly friends, but I was aware of his attraction to me. One night he asked me to a party at the nearby RAF camp. I agreed to go but never did reach the party. He took me to his room on the pretext that he wanted to collect his coat. Once inside the door he pounced on me, forcing me backwards on to a narrow bed on one side of the tiny room.

My skirt had been pulled up but I was fighting desperately to keep my knickers on and yelling for help. 'If you don't let me put it up your cunt I'll stick it up your backside,' he grunted. I resisted every attempt he made to penetrate me but knew he was getting more and more enraged. When he grabbed me round the throat with both hands I thought I was going to die and lay quite still hoping he'd think I was already unconscious. He got up and threw me on to the floor. I landed closer to the door than he was and knew I had to move fast if I was to get away. I scrambled up and was out of the door so quick, I didn't know if he was behind me or not. Down empty corridors I ran, screaming at the top of my voice.

A man came out of a room dressed only in a towel. He said he'd heard the screams but thought it must have been a joke. I pleaded with him to take me home. I stood in the doorway as he went back into his room to get dressed and only then noticed the other man lying on the bed, his body half-covered by the bedclothes. Both men spoke reassuringly to me and, once dressed, the man who'd been wearing the towel drove me home. Still upset and shaken by what had happened, I realized I was also very angry and decided I wanted to go to the police.

My statement took hours to write up because there were so many questions to answer and I was made to repeat each answer many times. One detective would ask by which arm the man had pulled me into the room and then another detective would ask the same question, followed by a third and a fourth detective, each of them repeating the question in exactly the same way. I quivered with humiliation throughout the whole ordeal and felt in a swirl of confusion and distress. Naively I'd believed I'd only have to tell my story simply and then the police would go and arrest my attacker. My anger kept me there, for I felt certain that I had the right to speak about what had been done to me. That man had almost killed me. I wasn't going to let him get away with it. I knew I was telling the truth, and, in the end, so did the police. They went to the barracks, found out that there was a party going on and arrested the man who'd attacked me. It was hard for me to take in that he could violently attack me and then go off to a party afterwards as though nothing had happened. He was held on remand until the court case some six months later. He pleaded guilty. Charged with attempted manslaughter, he was sentenced to eighteen months in prison.

I had not been called as a witness, so learned the outcome of the case when a detective phoned me at work. I remember my feelings were a tangle of different emotions as I thought about it all. Mostly I was relieved that it was over and done with; somebody had done something this time at least. I would imagine the court scene again and again, and wished I'd been there to see the look on his face when he'd been sentenced. In an odd way the outcome of that experience made me feel better about myself.

I'd become fearful of sex, fearful of becoming close to any man, until at nineteen I met Freddy. Those first six months we argued frequently about sex. He wanted us to deepen the relationship and I resisted. He was nine years older and that might have been a factor in feeling safe enough with him, eventually, to go ahead. Penetration was painful to begin with but I learned to trust him. Sex felt safe with him and, though I didn't orgasm much, it became pleasurable. But it took longer to realize I didn't love him. Three years later I ended the relationship, tormented by guilt and compassion, my self-esteem very low.

I drifted in and out of relationships, mostly with men who had other partners. On reflection, these were relationships that didn't require loyalty or commitment. I was living in a bed-sit at the time and as many of my friends were becoming involved seriously in long-term relationships, I saw less and less of them. Isolated and increasingly vulnerable, I felt unable to 'connect' with people.

I met John through a friend. He was four years younger than me and I thought he was a bit naive. He said he'd never met anyone like me before. What he meant was that I lived away from home, had a measure of independence and, well, was therefore more accessible for sex, wasn't I? Within three months I was pregnant and my life changed completely.

We moved into a flat and my isolation intensified. I didn't enjoy being pregnant, watching the changing shape of my body, beyond my control. It was a difficult and painful experience. I was convinced I looked horrendous – John stopped having baths with me and that only reinforced feelings of being ugly and unlovable. I didn't think or act. Instead I just allowed things to happen. This was my life, I reasoned; I was doing what every other woman did, settling down and having a child. I couldn't see beyond that.

Seven months into the pregnancy John announced that he didn't want the baby and suggested adoption. Not yet knowing my own mind I contacted a social worker and began going through the adoption process. I felt detached yet at the same time aware of this baby growing inside me. When the birth happened I had to have a Caesarean, and only the day before my discharge from hospital did I finally know what was right for me. I decided to keep my son and I called him Billy. It was the most important decision I'd ever made and even now symbolizes a significant change. Moving away from passivity and taking control of our lives can take a long while, but this decision and the implications involved meant that I'd begun that process.

John stuck around but remained ambivalent. We were together four years. During that time I came to realize that living with him was repeating the pattern of living with my father in that he would try to control and repress me and I would rebel in the same way as I had done when I was a child. As for the real issues, we would dance around them, only every confronting them in blazing rows. This growing perception was to have a profound effect on my thinking, making me connect with feelings I hadn't been in touch with, from my experience of abuse. There came a point when I had to face life head on and not push away the knowledge of the past. Further realizations and insights followed when a friend bought me a copy of Marilyn French's book *The Women's Room*, and later took me along to a women's group. I'd been introduced to feminism, and the connections I was now able to make taught me not only about my own life but about how common were the experiences of women in their relationships with men.

At one of those women's group meetings I met Linda. We'd known each other previously but had lost touch over the years. We were delighted to see each other again and renewed our friendship with excitement and interest. We became very close. Linda was confused about her sexual identity. She would have sex with men and then tell them she was a lesbian. I didn't understand, but then neither did Linda at the time.

There was definitely a sexual charge to our relationship – we would play-fight in a way that was obviously sexual, and it seemed natural for us to be intimate, to stroke, kiss and fondle each other. I was exploring with my body rather than with my mind. At one point Linda told me she wanted to have sex with me, at which I felt scared and threatened – I realized that I didn't really fancy her and that to go ahead would change our relationship irrevocably. I refused, and we never talked about it again. Then Linda stopped having sex with men; she knew she was a lesbian she said, but didn't know what to do about it. As there were/are no rules about how to come out, we spent long hours discussing what we could do. Despite the openness of the times and a growing awareness of choice, there were no guidelines to follow, no easy way of learning how to be more knowledgeable about the expression of sexuality.

The discussions in the group about sexuality had presented me with an alternative to heterosexuality. It was like finding a valuable piece of information, another piece of the jigsaw, something that could be a part of me, something real. The power of this new information exploded inside my head – 'blowing my mind' was an accurate description. I became separatist in outlook and totally rejected men. John was still around, still living with Billy and me, but his role in my life was no longer central. I was taking time out to think about things. There was so much going on that thinking was not so much a quiet time of reflection as a constant buzz of activity as new and amazing things were talked about, and I sampled and tasted and buzzed around for more. So much was happening: learning about feminism, developing my friendship with Linda and the growing understanding that I was attracted to women. I'd be sitting in a pub with friends when suddenly I'd see a woman I really fancied. My whole body would feel on fire and I wouldn't know what to do with myself. I had always found it easy to be cool and confident in similar situations with men – in any case, I always assumed they were thinking through their penises, no matter what. So I had never experienced that hot flushed feeling before and now it just bowled me over. It seemed both absurd and scary, not knowing how to proceed. Couldn't I have a normal conversation with this woman? Couldn't I act natural and just let things unfold without all this hot flushing and tongue-tied paralysis?

Linda and I would share our feelings about situations like this. My relationship with her was a stepping stone, part of a process enabling me to strengthen my sexual identity. I remember having a dream about that time and, while I didn't understand it then, I've never forgotten it. I was a man in the dream, being chased by the police because I had just murdered someone. Running into a hotel, I disguised myself as a woman and booked a room. The police were in the hotel looking for me while I was in the bar having a drink. I chatted up a man quite easily and took him to my room. He knew I was a man because he stroked my penis once we were on the bed.

Despite the care and support between Linda and me, once she came out as a lesbian, she began to withdraw from me. She decided to start up a lesbian-only group. I wanted to be involved but, of course, I wasn't a lesbian so I couldn't join. I felt totally rejected and could not understand the politics behind it all. When I spoke to Linda about it she would respond by getting very angry with me. Soon she'd met a woman she wanted to live with and I felt pushed more and more into the background of her past.

One evening I went to see her. I wanted to talk about our friendship and what we could do to rectify matters. She accused me of being jealous. We disagreed over a number of issues and our friendship ended on that note. I felt a great deal of hurt and pain over the loss of the relationship. Now I see that it would have ended sooner or later in any case.

Meanwhile things were deteriorating at home. John became intolerable, often forcing me to have sex. When I found out I was pregnant again it freaked me out completely. This time I decided on an abortion. Done on the NHS, it was a nightmare from start to finish. The doctors agreed that an induced abortion was best even though I was only twelve weeks pregnant. The nursing staff were judgmental and uncaring. I was discharged from the hospital with no arrangements made to get me home, and I lived some fifteen miles away. I don't know how long the journey took but I caught two buses and then a taxi, and once in the front door I collapsed.

Ill for about a month, I knew something had to be done about John and me once I recovered. I told him I couldn't go on as we were and, realizing it was all over between us, he became quite violent. More and more hostile as my growing independence became evident, he continued to force himself on me, wanting sex he said, but it was more like exerting a punishment. I took Billy and left the house, saw a lawyer, got a court injunction and he was ordered out of the house within a week. When Billy and I went back home all that was left in the house was Billy's bed. The whole affair was messy and stressful and the only thing that kept me going was hope for the future.

I'd been offered a place on a degree course at the local polytechnic. I was determined to build a new life for Billy and me. I looked forward to the years of study even though the immediate present was hard, living in a bare house with no money to replace what had been taken.

Nina and I met on the first day of the degree course. She had a child attending the polytechnic playgroup too. Nina was bright, academically sharper than me. But she didn't have much experience of life and would often contradict herself. She confided to me that she was a closet feminist and so I began talking to her about books and ideas and soon we were spending a lot of time together. Dissatisfied with a nearby women's group that we both thought was too 'middle class', we started up our own group at the poly, and became very active politically in student matters.

I realize in retrospect that without talking about it or even admitting it to ourselves, Nina and I had grown completely infatuated with each other. We spent almost all of our time together, except when she was having an affair with a man, when I would see little of her. We would stay overnight at each other's houses, often sharing a bed. One particular night Nina came on strong, saying that love-making between us would be 'an extension of our friendship'. The phrase grates on me these days as it can easily be misused. Naively I agreed, so long as there were no regrets afterwards. Nina was the first woman I had had sex with and, though we were both inexperienced, it aroused feelings I had never had with men. It was deeper and more bonding in some way, as well as more sensual. I wanted to explore further, but after the second time I stopped it. I realized that Nina had been using me, playing out a fantasy. It was a game to her. She refused to talk about it, nor would she discuss it at the CR group we both belonged to. Puzzled and hurt, I closed myself off from the idea of sex with women and soon afterwards became involved with a man.

Then things began to go very wrong. Nina became involved with a man twenty years older who had a reputation as a drug dealer. I tried not to think about it all and began talking more to Beatty, another CR group member. It took some time for things to come to a head and even now I am hazy about what happened when, but when Nina finished up being lovers with Beatty, I again felt great pain, confusion and concern as to what I should be learning from all this. I lost my friendship with both Nina and Beatty. Again I felt pushed to the outside of a situation I had once been an intimate part of. I had rejected Nina, but mainly because she had first rejected and used me. Learning how sexuality can be used destructively has been a harsh lesson for me, and it seems I've been learning that lesson all my life.

My reaction to what had happened was to throw myself into whatever relationships came along. I recognize now that I was using sex as a means of gaining affection – some kind of affirmation. Either I would be distant and indifferent, very much in control, or I would be running around like a headless chicken catering to everyone's needs but my own. I have always been attracted to relationships with problems; I have always thought I could resolve the problems by being that unique person who would be strong enough and caring enough to change the other individual. It soon became a pattern, with every new relationship having more difficulties than the one before (it culminated in living with a heroin addict). I would throw myself into it – it would be exciting, a challenge, I would give so much of myself, I would be stretched to my limits – and then end up burnt out and hurting. Later I realized that I was creating a painful dependency in the other person out of my own need to feel needed. The end of these relationships would arrive when, for whatever reason, I would suddenly decide I wanted independence.

It was a scary time and I felt my head was in bits. I had no centre or identity to draw on. How much I was aware of what was happening to me I can't really say – I have an ability to put things on hold and not question closely what I'm doing. It's a mechanism I learned as a means of survival, but which became a pattern for living. Even now, I suspend thinking about certain things I can't deal with and then bring them to the fore when I feel ready to sort them out.

After finishing my degree I undertook a course of therapy which lasted fourteen months. It gave me a lot more insight into myself and helped me understand some of the things that had happened to me. I can say now that it empowered me; it is thanks to that course that I have become the woman I am today.

My sexuality is an issue for me now – I go through phases where it seems to take up all of my thinking time. Most important is a growing awareness of the difference between the way I relate to women and the way I relate to men – a growing sense of the lesbian side of myself. Sometimes I feel very sure of myself; at other times I'm filled with doubts and denials.

My view of a sex life is very much in the abstract, except for masturbation. But being celibate helps me to focus and to take things slowly without the distraction a relationship would entail. I have the sense that through this period of calm, in which I'm putting my own needs first, I'm beginning to heal myself from a lifetime of destructive relationships. I am convinced that one day the right opportunity will come and I will meet a woman with whom I can express myself emotionally and sexually.

I know that my attraction to women was there from earliest childhood. I always had special girlfriends whom I loved and was in love with. The sexual games I played as a young child were always with other girls and always initiated by me. I remember once a friend doing a handstand with no knickers on. I got a real thrill out of it; I've never forgotten the feeling. It's a sensation I've recaptured with women, but never with men. I suppose in retrospect that I embraced heterosexuality because I wasn't aware of any other choice. Though my mother had told me not to trust men, there were no messages about loving women. A stable heterosexual relationship was the lifestyle to aspire to.

Obviously my experiences of abuse and rape could lead to the interpretation that I was, or am, rejecting men because of the violent harm they've done me. For a period of my life this was the case, but it was more a process I needed to go through to reclaim the power they had taken from me. Now I find men can be beautiful, sensitive and sexually alluring, as can women. My desire to explore my lesbian side is a positive drive, not a question of having rejected men and settling for second best.

Yet I also feel apprehensive, partly because of my lack of experience and partly because I suspect that with a woman there would be less room for pretence, for keeping a part of me separate. I know, too, that with a woman I would have to put myself in the position of learning a new language, new rituals, new codes of behaviour. It is difficult at thirty-five with the experiences I've had, to return to that position of bewilderment and powerlessness.

One of the things that frightens me at the moment about the idea of having a relationship with either a man or a woman is the idea of commitment. I want to hold back, or at least to keep a bit of myself back. I'm not sure that I trust myself, yet I know I will never find out unless I'm prepared to try. There are times when I feel lonely and long for companionship; on the other hand, life on my own, with my son, is so simple and I enjoy being selfish, something I haven't allowed myself for years. When I hear friends describing their relationships and listen to the games they play I feel determined never to get into that kind of situation again, idealistic as this might sound.

The knowledge I have gained from this period of celibacy, of focusing on myself rather than on anyone else's needs, is that I am no longer a victim. Writing this article has been part of that process.

Making sense of my memories
Grace Walker

When I was eight years old I was raped by a white man. I choose to call his actions rape, although he left me physically, if not mentally, intact. He was disturbed just as he was in the act of penetration, and the huge, sick guilt feeling I carry is that I wish he had gone ahead and finished the job. He raped me of everything else – my sexual innocence, my childhood. Perhaps if he had not been disturbed, if the whole event had happened, then I would be able to pack it away neatly into a dusty corner of my memory. This is exactly what I try to do. But, fourteen years later, I still freeze at the same point whenever I have sex – the point where that man was about to rape me. Love-making is far from lovely when this happens – it feels more as though I'm being reamed with a hoe. For me, the first time is every time. I would gladly forget the whole event. But I have no control over my memory. That man has been in my bed for fourteen years and I just don't know how to get him out.

My earliest and most vivid memory is, thankfully, a very happy one. When I was five years old I gained legal possession of a permanent and very caring family. I can consciously remember nothing before that time, which is odd since that same family had fostered me for the previous three years. It's as if my life began on that day. The adoption took place in the court-house of my Dorset home town. I can remember sitting, engulfed in a cold leather chair, and staring at the grey-faced magistrate. I can't remember his actual words, but I knew that I was the most important person in the room and the shaking of hands signified the end to a successful and important transaction. The best part of the whole event, however, was the sight of the new name on my school books – the same surname as my brothers and sister. The books were proof to anyone who dared to doubt my rightful place within this family.

With my coffee-coloured skin and jet-black hair I certainly stood out from the rest of my white family, so there were plenty of people who questioned, or worse, whispered about my origins. But my colour was, in those early days, a complexity more to those around me than to myself. After my adoption I felt special, happy in the knowledge that my parents had chosen me over anyone else to be their new daughter. My colour was simply a part of that 'specialness' – and for a short time I had a definite sense of pride in my brown skin and enigmatic past.

These were, of course, only feelings – my actual history was entirely unoriginal. I was born 'illegitimately', and my mother is half black. My father was either an Englishman or an Arab; she refused to say which. My mother had spent her whole childhood in a children's home, one of the many 'war babies' who were, supposedly, difficult to place with families of their colour. As she grew up she went from one unstable relationship to another, and when she became pregnant with me she realized that my only future lay with a family who could support me. She already had one son, my natural brother, who she had also placed in a home, but with whom she has always maintained contact. I have always felt rather jealous about this, but I realized long ago that there is nothing I can do – my mother refused to have any contact with me, and I now respect that decision.

I was two months old when my mother surrendered me to a children's home. They, in turn, fostered me out to several families until I was chosen by my parents. Denying my existence from the moment she gave me up was my mother's way of dealing with her decision, but she was so successful in her delusion that she would not sign the adoption papers for a child that she believed did not exist. I was five years old before she finally signed them, and – ironically – I was then lost to her forever. I often wonder how those five years must have seemed to her, desperately trying to forget her baby, yet constantly being plagued by the law that told her she was still not rid of me. Was it like living with a ghost? She's only a ghost to me. And is she ever curious about me? Because I remain so curious about her.

Being separated from that mysterious woman from such an early age meant that I had no conscious memory of her voice, or her touch. However, over many years the face of a woman would occasionally float in and out of my dreams, never speaking and never as a part of any dream sequence. She would simply appear, misty and ghostlike, and then fade away when I tried to focus on her. She had a large, round brown face and her hair was very dark and curly. I could never understand the mixed feeling of warmth and desperation I felt whenever she came into my dreams, and it wasn't until I saw a picture of my mother for the first time that I recognized this 'sleep-woman'.

The warmth of my originality and enigma soon wore off. The early glow of colour pride tarnished, so that by the time schooldays were over I felt very ashamed of my colour – a thing that I am only now transcending. There I was, five years old and brown-skinned, in a small school in Dorset which was a sea of hostile whiteness. I remember one little black boy who stayed at our school for a few weeks before returning home to Africa. He had no real knowledge of English so he used to repeat what the other children said. Consequently, out of ignorance rather than spite, he used to call me 'woolah' and 'blackie' along with the others. Perhaps because he was tougher than me, or more likely because children derive no pleasure in taunting someone who doesn't understand them, I never saw him receive any of the racist abuse that I received. He seemed to fit in as well as possible. But then I wouldn't have had time to notice if he had been receiving abuse, because I was too busy defending myself. It was odd to hear the word 'blackie' coming from someone who was so much darker than myself, and it makes me feel a bit sad to think of him being carried along with all the other kids. I hope that, wherever he is now, he's standing tall and proud.

I did, of course, have some friends. I lived in a typical suburban street overrun by scabby-kneed kids. But, with not one exception, every one of my friends turned to abuse me at some point or another. I don't feel any real animosity at this, however – not out of forgiveness, but because I wanted to fit in just like any other child. Had there been an object for my scorn, and thus a guarantee of my place in the gang, I perhaps would have taken advantage.

Outside school I used to keep away from the name calling, the taunting, by sticking around my sixteen-year-old sister. She used to help out at a local youth-club disco and occasionally I was allowed to go with her. One time there was this bloke who had been trying unsuccessfully to flirt with my sister and draw her attention. She had expressed her scorn in – knowing my sister – very graphic terms, so he turned his attention on to me, no doubt trying to revenge himself on my sister. I was, I suppose, rather flattered by the attentions of this grown-up 'boyfriend', as he called himself. After dancing with me, and parading me in front of my sister, he took me outside into the darkness. As he led me behind the women's toilets I heard the sound of Abba singing 'Waterloo' back in the disco. I vividly remember the strains of the song as he undid his, and my, trousers. His penis seemed enormous, with a revoltingly huge head. But I don't recall feeling scared when he first made me touch it, just rather repulsed by its warm dampness. I am haunted by a horrid fear that perhaps I wasn't as innocent as I think I was, even though I now understand that I have no reason at all to feel guilty. How is an eight-year-old supposed to know she's in danger from a man who's being 'nice' to her? He wasn't violent – just very persuasive in making me do things I don't want to put down on paper because that will make them harder to forget.

As he lay down and told me to take off my trousers I think maybe I began to wonder if this was bad, but I did as he said. He was in the process of pulling my body down on to his when I heard my sister call from around the corner. Then I definitely grew scared. I don't think I was before. But then, I was never scared of spiders until someone told me that they were scary.

While I ran back to my sister the bloke must have drifted into the darkness. It only occurs to me now that the whole event must have happened inside the space of about twenty minutes, though in my head it feels as though hours passed before my sister called. It's like a slow-motion piece out of some sick movie. My sister took in the sight of my ruffled clothes and 'caught red-handed' expression. All she said was, 'Don't you dare tell Dad.' I thought that this confirmed my guilt, but she knew then what I know now – that my father would have been jailed for that man.

From then on I realized that boys, and one girl, actually wanted that small part of me I kept hidden away in my knickers, and that any one of them would be my friend for such a seemingly small price. So, deriving no sexual pleasure whatsoever from the amateur fumblings of those pre-pubescent bouts, I whored for friendship because, outside school, I had no packed lunch to give. I came to realize that the moment my knickers were back up I was relegated again to my status as 'black blur' or 'choc-ice', but for that small moment I could revel in my dubious popularity. Such was my ignorance (no longer innocence, there wasn't much innocence in my actions) and desperation, I gratuitously exploited myself for reasons which, at that age, seemed perfectly logical.

By fourteen those sexual interchanges had all but tailed off, and I was still physically intact. To those boys I suppose I was the first rung on the sexual ladder – and I certainly was trodden on. But they moved on to more serious fucking with far more socially 'acceptable' girls. The one girl with whom I shared my lunch and myself recently married.

Secondary school was unbearable. *They* (most of the pupils and some of the teachers) had finally succeeded in making me hate myself, although I understand now that my extra-curricular activities did nothing to enhance my feelings of self-respect. I began to understand, and detest, a system that forced me to sit in the same classroom as people who hissed 'Go home wog' at me, and vandalised my desk and workbooks with racist graffiti – a system that expected me to gain a useful education from a teacher who told me to 'get back where I came from'.

The worst time was from my fourteenth to sixteenth years, because I was starting to wake up to the fact that I was never going to change colour, and that I would have to look forward to this kind of abuse for the rest of my life. The reason why I received so much of it lay, I think, in my lack of defence, my indefinable ethnicity. I'm not, to many people, black enough to be called black, nor am I white enough to be called white. Consequently, on the rare occasions when I would bother to complain, the answer I received was the dubious palliative of 'But you're not even *black*' – which is, of course, as racist as the abuse itself.

After countless physical attacks I learnt how to 'fight dirty', but on one occasion no amount of dirty fighting defended me from the aggression of a woman of twenty-odd. She had been offended by my refusal to apologize to *her* for pushing *me* from the kerb and insulting me. I took such a battering that I had to explain to my mum why I had arrived home bruised and bleeding from a wound on my head where the woman had pulled a patch of hair from my scalp. Before this I had never bothered to complain, rightly believing that my parents could do very little. But this time they whisked me off to the police station. They were faced with a frighteningly 'laid back' attitude, and told that it was probably 'six of one and half a dozen of the other – you know what kids are like'. When my dad pointed out that the woman lived near my school and that I knew her name, the officer simply presented my dad with her address. He then suggested my dad go and 'have a few words with her'. This typical small-town policeman was too busy, or rather too scared, to bother about a little bit of racial harassment in a place with a vast white majority. Their attitude can easily be summed up: 'Let the wog-bashers carry on – so long as we don't have to worry our provincial little heads about it.'

By sixteen I had largely given up on school, although I was forever being told that I 'could do better'. Doing no work meant more time for other things. I was having half-hearted sex with a boy down the road, despite being rather bored with the whole scene by now. He was being nice to me – so why not just carry on? – even though he wouldn't acknowledge me in public or announce me as his girlfriend. I stupidly told myself it was because he was shy. Just after my sixteenth birthday we decided to go 'all the way'. My strongest feeling was one of mortifying embarrassment as he repeatedly tried to enter me – heightened by his frustrated whispers of 'relax, you're too tight'. In the end he decided I was frigid, and so we ended whatever it was that we'd had.

It's ironic that it wasn't until the very end of my school career that I struck up one of the most important relationships of my life. It was with a white woman who had been the head of my lower school when I was eleven or twelve, a time when I was coming to terms with a lot of things and was a very disruptive and anti-social member of the classroom. At that time, using a mixture of laughing, shouting, comforting and understanding, she had managed to save me from lapsing into criminal delinquency. I was sent to her when I was at my most unco-operative and sullen. She would take me by the hand and say, 'One day you are going to leave all of this, and you are going to *be* someone. You are a good person, never forget that.' She had, and still has, endless faith in me. At school, however, I never believed her, and even alienated myself from her because I was utterly convinced of my own unworthiness. But when I left school and all of its pressures behind, I began to respect myself much more, and to realize the importance of our friendship. So I made a concerted effort to try to start living up to her belief in me. Our friendship has grown over the years, to the point where we have an almost telepathic understanding of each other. I have never felt the need to tell her about my childhood, since I feel that she has some kind of a clue anyway. I see her very much as my guide and mentor, although I'm not sure how she sees me – except as a friend.

Leaving all the racism of school behind, I felt that I had, in a way, lost a part of myself. Before, I had had a racial identity forcibly bestowed on me, one that – however difficult it was – I could use as a defence. Now those who had dictated my identity were no longer around, because being in their company was not compulsory any more. I became obsessed with discovering my 'roots' and, with them, some kind of racial niche. I contacted the children's home from which I had been adopted, and saw the woman who had supervised my adoption. I discovered many seemingly trivial, but to me priceless, facts about myself, for instance my birth weight. I also found out that my father *was* an Arab. I was told that my mother maintains contact with the agency and that she lives and works in Greece, and does not want to be in contact with me. The counsellor gave me a photograph of her, and I was disappointed to see that we do not look very alike, perhaps I take after my father? But apparently my mother and I are alike in terms of personality – we share an irreverent sense of humour – and our voices are similar.

To describe every sexual encounter I've had over the past five years would prove to be long and very boring. Like most of my friends at college I had lots of short, and a couple of long, relationships with men, and a couple more with women. I used to fend off kind attempts by boyfriends to rid me of my virginity with tired old excuses like 'I'm not on the pill' or 'I'm allergic to rubber'. It was easier to make up excuses than to face their scorn or sympathy at my inexplicable tension when it came to penetration. Sex was fine up to that point though, and I developed my 'immature' clitoral orgasm to a fine art. So I continued to have boyfriends for however short a time, and my 'problem' didn't bother me much as long as I derived some pleasure out of sex.

But when I did at last fall in love I decided that I just could not let this man go, no matter what I had to do. He was, of course, the epitome of my romantic and lustful dreams – tall and handsome, proud and black – we were crazy about each other. Trusting him and wanting him as I did, I thought it best to tell him about my childhood experiences. It was the first time that I had told anyone because of the sense of shame I still carried. I half wish I had not, because it opened the door to the bitterness I had stored for many years. He was very sympathetic with me, including sexually. For a long time he did not pressure me and sex was good, at least it was for me. But after a while tension developed, and eventually we split up because he said he did not want to hurt me. I did not want this interminable hang-up of mine to ruin another relationship, so we got back together and, rather than lose him, I let him force me.

In the midst of the pain I could almost hear my sister's voice calling for me – only this time she was too late. I don't know why this moment of realization had not occurred until now – that every time I came near to penetrative sex I felt as though I was eight again, with the same feelings of guilt, disgust and, now, fear. Perhaps it was because I had told someone the whole story and this had made the link in my own mind between my present situation and the events in my childhood.

During all this my boyfriend was experiencing the disapproval of his staunchly Pan-Africanist friends, who were unhappy about our relationship on the simple grounds that I was not black enough. The threat of losing his friends was the key to his escape from our rapidly deteriorating relationship. Although his leaving at that point nearly sent me over the edge into a total breakdown, I am grateful that he never once alluded to my sexual situation as the real cause, although we both knew it was.

On my own I hit the booze and dope in a big way. It was easier to spend each day completely 'out of it' than to dwell on the past, which was too painful, or the present, which was too hard, or the future, which was too far away to contemplate. My coursework, which to date had been minimal, was now non-existent and so I had to go to see a counsellor who tried to put my mind back in order. What she succeeded in doing was to probe enough to have me in floods of drunken, hysterical tears and then tell me that she 'wasn't there to give answers' although she suggested I try seeing a sex-therapist. The one good thing she did do was to pull some strings and get me a transfer to a new college in a big city.

I spent a year in Sheffield, getting my act together and cleaning my system out, both mentally and physically. I made the choice to live alone – so I had the time and privacy to learn to live with myself. I think that I forged a new self during that year. In the cloying atmosphere of my old college I had rediscovered whole chunks of my past that needed to be dealt with, and here, in the anonymity of a large city, with time alone, I could find a way of coping with those memories.

One thing that had a profound effect upon my self-image was to see myself as a black person. I had, of course, always been very aware of my colour, but only in a negative way, as a response to others' racism. During that year I was given the opportunity to study a diverse selection of black literature. I reflected on the images of black people worldwide, and at a personal level. Until this time I had never really seen myself as 'universally' black, and I had never felt 'politically' black. Although I had been a member of an anti-racist group at my old college it was more as a sympathetic supporter than as an integral member, as a black woman. Finally, I realized that I was proud of my colour and, knowing where my 'roots' lie at least on one side, I developed a deep interest in Afro-American culture, an interest I'm still extending.

Not surprisingly, I felt a new kind of strength about my colour; but there was still a great deal of anger and humiliation over my sexuality, and this remains true today. My anger was not of the explosive kind; it throbbed beneath all my newly discovered colour pride, gently but profoundly. This anger was fuelled by a deep sense of self-disgust as I looked back over my childhood, which I perceived to have been dirtied by my early and enforced introduction to sex. I *knew* that this self-disgust and guilt at my own behaviour was unfounded – and that it was the disgust at what the man actually did to me that continued to make me freeze when making love.

My year of living alone and 'getting my act together' did not sort this out, but it did give me the chance to write about my experiences and, in doing so, to impose some form of order upon those chaotic and self-destructive thoughts that had been occupying my mind.

Drafting and redrafting this article has forced me to think hard about my perceptions of myself and my sexuality. I've had to ask myself what I really want out of life, and how I'm going to set about looking for an answer to my 'hang-ups'. Is writing for this book, perhaps, a part of that process? Writing, thinking, rewriting and rethinking has given me some answers to my questions. I do not now hope or expect a simple remedy to rid me of my guilt about the past. I realize that this feeling was unfounded – but facing it, rather than tucking it away deep in my memory, gives me a chance of ridding myself of that moment in my early life that still influences me now.

I neither hope nor expect to be swept off my feet by Mr Wonderful – or Ms Wonderful – not yet, anyway. After so many years of performing like some kind of pathetic clown jerked by other people's string pulling, the last thing I intend to do now is conform to any preconceived 'type'. What I'm saying is that I may get over my sexual 'problem' or I may not. At this moment I'm actually enjoying living with *myself*. I can suddenly see many of my good points. I feel fresh and hopeful for the future. I realize that there does not *have* to be a resolution to every story, at least not a traditional happy ending. But I feel great, after all these years – thanks to some close friends, thanks to putting it all down in writing, thanks to 'discovering' my colour. I actually *like* myself. It's as though I've found a new friend, and she will suit me perfectly for the moment.

Moving in, moving on
Alice Land

At this point in my life I am choosing not to be in an intimate relationship. Because, fundamentally, I am content and satisfied on my own. And because there is not enough room in my life for a relationship. And because I still feel so damaged emotionally from my childhood, I know if I choose a relationship again it will reflect that unresolved damage. I want to explore my history and to heal those wounds, to become more whole, and then maybe ...

My ancestors on both sides are wandering Jews. My family has been moved on countless times over the centuries – the Spanish inquisition, the Russian pogroms, Nasser's Egypt ... these are the stories I know. Each time, whether rich or poor, we have picked ourselves up and headed off to another country, another life. My family has its roots in every other country in the world.

I think that wandering is in my blood – a compulsive inner drive that says 'don't settle yet', or 'watch out', or 'are you sure?'. For most of my young adulthood I owned only what I could carry in one carload of black plastic bags. I camped in many places and moved on every few months, eagerly, excitedly, never putting down roots, delighting in making each new home. It has been the same with my intimate sexual relationships, the moving on, that is. I move in, either literally or metaphorically, and then sooner or later I go. Sometimes I am beaten to the going stage.

My inner childhood was a desert. I have so few memories, just every now and then an oasis, a richness of colour so bright it hurts. The rest is masses of nothingness, a great inner loneliness so well armoured that it rarely showed. I'm told that when I was a child we moved a lot – London, Brighton,

Manchester, I don't know where else. Stories not told. My family just happened, it seems to me now.

My paternal grandparents had an old-fashioned arranged marriage. They liked each other when they married, then respect grew, and more liking, and then a love so strong it lasted a lifetime. My grandfather, a self-made man, became rich enough to educate his eldest son at an English public school. Born and brought up in Egypt, a small, dark-skinned (mostly from freckles), foreign boy, my father was sent to England by boat on his own at the age of eight. He suffered horribly – the cold, the food, the beatings, the bullying, the teasing, emotional deprivation, ill health, and so on. He went home only for the summer holidays.

My father became a supremely critical, dictatorial man who laid down the law on everything that happened in the family. There was only one way: his way. His obsession with cleanliness and tidiness made our lives hell. We had to eat without making any noise and eat what we asked for – we weren't allowed to make a mistake and if we couldn't finish it would be dished up to us at the next meal. I was forever scrubbing my nails, they never came up to scratch.

It was not that he didn't feel affection, he just couldn't show it, he told me many years later. I felt suddenly so sad, I didn't know for a moment for whom – for him for being so damaged, or for the small child in me who felt so unloved.

My mother's family is English working class, peasant stock with an injection two or three generations back of Russian or German Jews. Of these ancestors I know virtually nothing. I remember making bread with my maternal grandfather and letting it rise by the coal fire, eating unlimited forbidden foods (cakes, salty butter melting in the plate, roast dinners), sleeping on the lumpy sofa by the fire's last glow, sipping sweet tea from a saucer with cuddles and laughter in the early morning. I knew without a doubt from these grandparents that I was loved and that I was lovable, that I was OK. I planted this seed of OKness deep in my centre and it took root so strongly that throughout my life, no matter how rough or awful the times, I have always been able to know that deep down, I am OK.

My grandmother struggled to bring up her five children mostly on her own, so it was the eldest, my mother, who gave up her childhood to mother her sisters and brother. She was saved by the war, which allowed her to leave home and taste independence. Then she met my father. I don't know if they were ever really happy together beyond the falling in love stage, beyond the honeymoon. The early years deprived of parenting showed up in my mother when she had her own children. Her love and affection were tainted by fear and depression. She just wasn't happy. Her ability to tolerate conflict was so low that if my brother and I argued she would threaten to kill herself. Her unhappiness stuck like syrup to much of my childhood and dripped over our family psyche so that as a teenager I longed for her death. Small needy children were a pain for her. She wanted us to be her friends. I didn't like sweets as a child.

My mother never let a week go by without moving a piece of furniture. Nothing was allowed to take root. To this day she moves house as often as is decent and if she can't move house she re-papers walls, fiddles with the furnishings or moves the pictures around. In the garden every plant and shrub, however large or small, is in constant danger of being moved on. As for my father's family, there is not one close to me who is married or even in a live-in relationship, though some have been married, some more than once, and some have had children.

I remember my only brother with mixed feelings. We fought a lot – he was good, I was bad. He kept his room tidy, his fingernails clean, and saved his money. I couldn't. We had brief truces, my brother and I, but basically I knew he was on the side of my parents and I have not forgiven him.

When I was fifteen my parents separated. My father waved goodbye to us from the front porch and I felt a sharp, tearing pain in my chest as my mother and brother and I drove away. My heart broke. Until that moment I had hated him, had been desperate to leave. I grew up fast in that moment and made up a story about my life: that nothing is permanent and I would never expect it to be. I understood that since relationships do not last I would never expect them to. I promised myself that I would never show my heart.

My sexuality has been shaped by strange experiences, by feelings so powerful they could not be ignored, and by mixed messages.

There was my friendship with Rachel, at age eight. She lived in total chaos with her liberal parents. She wanted to be me, to have the order, the carpets and the central heating, and I wanted to be her – the terrible mess and dirt everywhere, the freedom. We were both emotionally neglected by immature, damaged parents. We were bonded by loneliness and by sensuality. We loved to touch, spent ages at night stroking each other's backs. We read precociously and under the covers – the 'dirty' parts of *Lady Chatterly's Lover* and *Fanny Hill*. I learned to enjoy being physically close to another person, learned that touch is delicious and touching gives great pleasure.

Later, as an adolescent, there was a girlfriend with whom I started to explode with sexual feelings so powerful I didn't know where to put them. We played a tying-up game after taking off some of our clothes. I remember a hot summer's day with the curtains closed wickedly against the light. Enormous excitement. We never talked about this event. I assumed it was not OK.

I was also intellectually curious. I found a book on my father's shelf – *The Psychology of Sex* – an ancient and worthy leatherbound tome. I found out that women who masturbate become insane. I was very frightened. I didn't realize at the time that it was only the insane women who were crazy enough to be caught. I acted out my sexuality in secret and very quietly. I assumed that I was very bad, and that one day I would go mad.

I carried on masturbating and being turned on by the fantasies from that leatherbound tome. I remember at the age of perhaps six or seven going to the seaside, at six in the morning – we had to be first to miss the traffic and were there digging holes by eight. I remember driving there in our little car, an Austin 7, our post-war nuclear family. So was it boredom that led me to have the sexual fantasies? I'd sleep or pretend to sleep and while I pretended I would fantasize – wild, sadomasochistic sexual fantasies. I looked forward to night-time, when I would be able to masturbate. I masturbated every night (even when I had promised myself I wouldn't). And once I found my vagina I put things into it. Once a hair-grip got lost but it worked its way down eventually, much to my relief. I assumed that I was wicked, beyond redemption.

And then I remember being ill. With illness, whether a cold or an ear infection, I remember not being able to shit. Maybe it was because when I was sick I was force-fasted until the fever went down. For some reason I didn't lie about the shitting – perhaps I didn't dare to. In any case, I didn't mind about it, but my father did. I must have an enema. I remember being very young and lying on a cold bathroom floor naked from the waist down and being buggered by a plastic penis, very gently. It was for my own good. A healthy ejaculate pumped into my rectum. I felt hurt and shamed and violated. I felt a disgust so strong, so overwhelming that I wanted to die. I protested with silent tears and turned these feelings on myself. I had nowhere else to put them because I knew that my parents were right. They had told me over and over. Then I knew that I was disgusting. I felt then self-disgust and I could not bear to look at my genitals or my anus.

I read fairy stories and cookery books when I was ill. I learned to be healthy. I learned to be patient and silent. Now I take an active part in my waitings, but as a child my waiting was passive. I said to myself that one day I'd be free and then no one would tell me what to do. I counted the years and then I counted the months and then I counted the weeks and the days. My childhood was like a fucking prison sentence. I served my time. Nothing on this earth could entice me to relive my childhood.

I learned an inner pride. Because it was so difficult to protest and the punishments were so severe – emotional punishments, terrible silences, the withdrawal of communication, of warmth, of affection, of company – I preserved my inner integrity by saying nothing. But my thoughts were free. I mouthed my answers silently, the words I wasn't free to speak out loud. As an adult I fought with authority figures over and over until I understood the unconscious need in me to resolve my unexpressed anger towards my parents – for squashing me, for hating my laugh, for making approval conditional and love unattainable.

I developed stamina. I learned to bide my time. I imagined a wall around me to keep me safe. I still do at times. But then it made me invisible and isolated.

I learned an almost remarkable ability to adapt and cope, to be resourceful. I was not afraid to move on. I welcomed change.

I learned above all to be a survivor. I chose fierce independence. I became good at looking after myself.

When I was about sixteen my mother began to encourage me in strange ways to be promiscuous. She got me a job as a hostess in a men's nightclub by lying about my age. Sure, I had sex with some of them. Only once did it really feel like rape – I didn't want it, and said so, but I wasn't heard. My 'no's were very small then.

Then when I was seventeen she asked what I later discovered to be an ex-lover of hers to look after me when she went on holiday, because she didn't trust me on my own. I had sex with him. I felt bad, dirty bad, but I wanted it. I was desperate to find out and I didn't know how, other than by doing it. I thought that doing it would illuminate some dark corner of my life.

I remembered my first fuck two years earlier – a coldly calculated hour of sex. I expected something and was astonished and very puzzled by almost nothing. No feelings. I continued to be puzzled for many years. I knew that the feelings I got with masturbation were bad, and I expected something different with sex. I was in my twenties before I found out that an orgasm is an orgasm, however it comes.

My mother told me about the mechanics of sex, about the gynaecologist she knew who would do an abortion if ever I needed one. I don't remember any advice about contraception, about love, about relationships, about choices, about how to say yes and no appropriately. I felt I couldn't ask. I thought sex was a bad, secret thing. It was never talked about openly. I learned not to talk about it. For years I chose lovers who didn't talk, and I stayed ignorant.

This was the 1960s – so-called sexual freedom. I let my hair down all the way. I went into many relationships and moved on when they didn't work. Or they moved me on.

Over the years I absorbed a long list of mixed messages. These include: sex is bad, don't do it; deny, deny, sexual feelings don't exist; be secretive about sex; hide your body, stay thin, don't put on weight; sex is for making babies; sex and love come in separate packages; boys only want one thing;

don't ask for what you want; don't be forward; don't be noisy; don't make a spectacle of yourself; don't touch; don't ask; don't talk ... And so I have two opposing forces in my life – do it versus don't do it. Do it is sexual, physical, expressive and vital; don't do it is asexual, terrified, ashamed, small and mute.

I was very old at sixteen. One day I was ditched by a boy I loved totally and absolutely and I tried to kill myself. But in the act of trying to die I found out how much I wanted to live. It was at that moment that my real life began. A life of discovery and recovery.

I took my struggle to a psychotherapist. By that point I had a young child I loved, but I felt depressed a lot of the time. I decided not to repeat my mother's pattern of parenting, so I took my Pandora's box to my therapist and over a period of eight years I examined its contents. Each time I took something out, especially if that something was a sexual secret, I exposed myself with great trepidation and fear. Would this be it? Would I find out now that I was really a monster? Each time I heard 'You're OK.' And each time I healed a little more.

I fought the messages and the lies that I had gathered, that had poisoned me for so many years. It took so long. Now I am healing abuse – the abused and confused and neglected child, the humiliation, the degradation, the sexual abuse. Now I know it is my parents who behaved disgustingly (albeit unintentionally), but though I know this in my mind, the feelings their behaviour invoked, unexpressed through so many years, are laid down in all the cells of my body. They surface slowly, sometimes unexpectedly, always painfully. I heal these wounds by screaming and crying, by ranting and raving. And each time I release more memories, and with them more feelings, and I feel less small and powerless, more OK, more loving and accepting of myself. Only now do I feel good about my genitals.

It is through my work in psychotherapy that I have discovered how not to be a victim of my own inner needy child, how to grow up, how to respect myself, how to be more myself, how to choose to be visible. My anger enabled me to heal, it is the feeling that unlocked every door. My anger enabled me to feel the hurt and the shame and to cry. Initially it erupted like an errant firework, in unpredictable fits and starts. Now I am calmer and wiser.

I have successfully shaped a life which is rich and full – a flowering oasis. I feel fundamentally sane and healthy most of the time, and mostly unshakably happy. I have a deep-rooted passion for my child, my work and my close friends and a growing love of myself. These are my priorities.

I have learnt that being alone is not all bad. A relationship takes time, energy, commitment; I have not enough time left over. Besides, I am revelling in doing what I want to do when I want to do it. I have discovered the many joys – great and small – of being my own mistress. There is being able to talk for two hours at the end of the day to a dear friend on the phone; going to the movies five nights in a row; buying myself flowers; having a bath for as long as I like; not sharing my bed; not having to say no if I don't feel like making love; waking up in the mornings and remembering my dreams; being able to be a mother to my child without competition; eating only when I feel hungry. It is the beginning and the end of the day that I give to myself – precious times of nurture and creativity, rest and reflection, aimless pottering and mad impulses. I am increasingly protective of these times.

The relationship I have with my child is an ever-changing source of challenge and joy. He has talked about his hurt, about how much he hurt when his parents separated. The damage is done now. But at least we talk about our feelings and our mistakes.

My history has shaped me. As a mother I have struggled to find the mother within me, and still do. One day, when I have exorcised those parts of my own mother which I have unwittingly taken in, I will forgive my own mother. I am becoming more successful in not letting my son hear the cries of the needy child within me.

I have made myself a home with strong roots. This frightens me, because it makes me feel vulnerable. For the first time I do not want to move on. I feel a softening inside. Sometimes I move around at night and look for different places to sleep. Sure, I make an excuse – this room is too cold or too hot, the bed is too hard or too soft. But I look forward to when a storm brews and I pile cushions by the fire and curl up under the duvet with my child and my dog.

In most areas of my life I feel strong: I know who I am and what I want. I am reliable, I have integrity, I feel respected and loved. But my personal sense of entitlement doesn't extend very far beyond me – I am the oasis – I have created all that I need within me. I am almost totally self-sufficient. Almost – thank god. I know I won't always live like this; I look forward to sharing my life one day, when I am ready. I know that one day I will find a relationship that suits both the nomad and the stay-at-home that I am growing into.

Inevitably, my life has moved on again since I wrote this chapter. But that's another story ...

All about labels
Halima

My identity is still developing, even though I am a supposedly sexually mature woman in my early thirties, married with three children. I say I am still finding out who I am because I feel that the labels attached to me from the day I was born – black, working class, female, pretty – have charted my life and I am still trying to analyse how far society has shaped who and what I am today. Being of mixed parentage, a black Somali father and white British mother, with two diverse religions, Muslim and Christian, two cultures that are worlds apart, I know all about labels. As a friend once said, first we were half-caste, then coloured, and now we are black.

A lot of the problems I experienced in adolescence were caused by the contradictions between the different cultures my parents came from. For example, in my father's culture polygamy – marriage to two or more women – was the norm. He comes from a nomadic tradition in which infant mortality is high and life-expectancy low. Therefore reproduction is very important. Also important is the value placed on a male child, who can marry outside the tribe, thereby extending it and acquiring more cattle. These are customs that to British people like my mother appear sexist and adulterous. So my mother used to criticise my father for things that were simply part of his culture – his habit of tying his luggage up with string or his lack of ability when it came to painting and decorating the house. She never thought to take into account that nomads have homes constructed from rushes that can be transported on the backs of camels, so what would he know about bricks and mortar? We children witnessed terrible arguments between them. Usually it was my mother who won.

I was never close to either of my parents. I would have loved a closer bond with my mother; by contrast, I would have preferred to be a million miles away from my father. He was an alcoholic and a seaman. When I was a child he meant trouble and I used to dread the telegram that would proclaim his arrival home. It would be delivered by motorbike and if I was playing in the street the roar of a passing motorbike would always distract me. After years of fighting with him my mother found it extremely difficult to show any affection. She had an outer shell as cold and tough as steel and even during the most traumatic episodes with him she would never cry.

My mother interpreted the problem between herself and my father as one of colour. Like so many white people, she made the assumption that all black people possessed the disadvantages of the individual she happened to know. As a child I found her views very confusing. If he was bad, were all black people like him? Was I? Or if this applied only to men, what about my brothers? I knew that they weren't bad, but how did other white people see them?

I felt deeply responsible for my mother's plight. Here she was, a beautiful white woman who had met and fallen in love with a black man. For this she had been ostracized by her family and even when times were bad she knew she could never go back because she would have been unable to take us children, blatant proof of that relationship, with her. Later I reacted against my mother for the pain she caused me. In telling me black men were no good it was as if the whole race was written off in one stroke. Because I was black myself I came to feel betrayed. And this betrayal developed into a sense of affinity with black men, with people who were judged by the colour of their skin rather than by their personality or character.

Physically I didn't fit the black stereotype. I had straight hair, a light skin colour and European features. Black kids used to call me 'Paki' and whites used to compliment me on how nearly white I was. But I was proud of my Somali heritage and wanted other people to know about it. I wanted desperately to look black, to have an Afro. When I was very young I had wanted to meet a rich white man; later I rebelled against my mother and it was black youths I felt easy with. I longed to meet a Mr Right who would be all the things my father was not.

I know my mother had had bad experiences, but the problem was that she never explained them: only the feelings of distrust were transmitted to me. I often wish she could have sat down with me and related her past history, both the negative and positive aspects of her relationship, so I could have formulated my own opinions. Her experience with my father led her to dismiss all men as animals. I was taught that men lied, cheated and were only interested in one thing: sex. I found this very confusing and wondered who would ever be interested in me.

Yet in other ways my mother had been training me for my gender role since birth. She saw me as a tomboy and tried to counteract this by making me do a lot of the domestic work. When it came to education, my sisters and I had no choice but to leave school because of economic pressures from which my brothers were protected. We went to work in factories to support their university education. My mother felt it was important to give my brothers their freedom; they were emancipated from poverty at the cost of our oppression and imprisonment in a life of boredom.

It is unpleasant and even painful to look back at my adolescence. They say time heals, but I don't believe that. My early sense of my sexuality involved getting crushes on boys, my mother being dragged in by my father, the arguments between them, hearing my father, in an effort to break down my mother's moral superiority, say that I'd end up a prostitute on a street corner. I wasn't allowed to have relationships with boys and reacted against my father for forcing my mother to make my life so hard. It was easy to blame him for everything she did.

My awareness of myself as a sexual being first dawned on me when people began to react differently to me. I was aware of the physical effect I had on certain people around me and I couldn't understand it. Sexuality was power to my adolescent mind, an awareness of the value of mascara-weighted eyes, the provocative wiggle which I knew was a 'turn-on' without understanding why. My life became strange and exciting – the whispered secrets I shared with friends, a sense of belonging to my own sex. Then there was being noticed by boys, who would demand either by kindness or cruelty that I notice them in return. I found I was no longer included in the football matches at the corner of the street and missed the taste of cool fresh water out of pop bottles at half-time. Now I was either a water-carrier or a distant observer.

Menstruation marked a number of changes in my life. It too was pleasure and pain. Sexuality at this point was about having to make toilet paper into a pad when I was having my period; rolling my long grey pleated skirt up above my knees; shaving my legs and under my arms when the hairs were hardly visible. It was shaping my eyebrows; wearing a 30AA bra bought from the catalogue; hiding the holes in my sisters' cast-off tights. I remember brushing my hair a hundred times to make it shine while at the same time being unable to take a bath or iron my clothes when I wanted because of the cost of electricity. Measuring up was of utmost importance. What size are you? She hasn't got any at all. Above all, I remember the pressure of it all – of being torn between loyalty to my mother's standards and the wish to conform to my friends' behaviour, of striving to find a place for myself as an individual within a conformist group.

Adolescence was a time of cryptic clues and phrases. Do you give? How far do you go? You have to be careful. They're all after one thing. The metamorphosis seemed to happen overnight: men became animals, girls became women, mothers became naggers, and I was a problem. Emotions came easy. Marvin Gaye made me cry. I had crushes and blushes. I hated my mum because she disliked me.

My friends at this time were both black and white. I saw no difference in our interests and views: the most significant thing was our relationship, the most superficial the colour of our skin. My two closest friends happened to be white. Carol was one of this pair: we were close all through secondary school and made plans to continue our friendship for ever. She lived in a white, middle-class suburban area; I lived in a predominantly black, inner-city area. My mother would reluctantly let me travel the miles to Carol's home, a stable haven that seemed worlds apart from my own, and sleep over. Two things in particular amazed me: the happy relationship between her parents, and her bedroom. Her mother and father would smile at each other and Carol's dressing-table was full of toiletries. Later I began to make a distinction between black and white friends and the importance of this distinction would lead me to part company with the whites I knew and to seek out only black friends. This was a crucial time in my life; these friends' seemingly insignificant actions shaped my future.

As a black woman I had a lot of problems in trying to conform to a feminine stereotype I did not fit into. This is where I think that my experience of racism has given me a deeper understanding of sexism. We black women have never been able to find ourselves in European images of women; growing up in Britain I didn't find any images of myself, nor could I identify with the few images of black women in the media or in my school books. So it was easy for me to understand that my white counterparts couldn't either. Today I consider myself a feminist, one who wears make-up for no one other than herself, perhaps as a shield to hide behind. In any case, make-up makes me feel more able to face the world, which is important to me.

I am married now to a black man and we have three children. I would say my relationship with both my husband and the children is good: I love my children and they know it. We are all able to talk openly together and as parents we take time and trouble to explain things to our children. My husband at times displays anxieties over our teenage son that jog memories of my own childhood, though his concern is more to do with the problems for a black youth of growing up in these times and the threatening environment we live in.

I have recently returned to full-time education. This has helped me in understanding the relationship between my parents and many of the problems I encountered in growing up. Through reading and having the opportunity to discuss issues that are important to me and my family I am gaining in self-confidence. I am beginning to feel good about myself.

... doin' it on my own
Pearlie McNeill

I was in my thirty-fifth year when I heard the word mentioned for the very first time. Masturbation. There it was, a label, a meaning, a connection, fitted on to my own life. Mas-tur-bation. So that's what it's called. To think there was a word for that activity of mine that was as familiar to me as washing my hair or making a bed. I looked around at the other faces in the group. The woman went on reading from a book about women's sexuality.

It was our Friday night meeting. I'd recently joined and was learning about feminism. Originally, I'd come to make known a self-help group that I was involved with, but something about the way these women discussed things drew me in. I was learning about important issues but with varying degrees of interest and reluctance.

I tried now to pay attention, to follow what was being said, but my mind had fastened on that word. I tasted the sound of it, rolling it silently around the inside of my mouth. I felt like a tolled bell; reverberating memories and questions tumbled around my head each time I repeated the word. Mas-turbation. Well, if there was a name for it then that meant ... I looked again at the relaxed faces, the warm smiles. Does that mean that they ...

I can't remember when I began masturbating but I do know the practice was well established by the time I was five or six. I cannot dredge up recollections of body exploration nor can I point to any person and say they initiated or encouraged me in the habit. It is simply there, a part of me, something that I did at frequent intervals from early childhood onwards. In my teen years I developed uneasy feelings about the need to satisfy myself in this manner but these feelings gave way when I realized finally that what I was doing with myself was better than going with boys.

My mother caught me twice when I was small. There I was sitting at the kitchen table, elbows dug firmly into the wooden top, while underneath, my legs were moving in a rotating fashion. I had no idea what I was doing, had never even touched myself 'down there' but my mother responded angrily. She called it *jibblajerks* and by her stern reprimand I learned it was *bad*. After being caught a second time a few months later I must have decided it was something to do when no one else was around. My mother had intended to convey disgust but somehow this message hovered above me rather than taking up residence inside and, with a need that was already strong, I responded to that and not to my mother's disgust. I'm still amazed I wasn't caught in later years, for the manner in which I chose to masturbate would certainly have provoked a strong reaction from my parents.

You see I had a particular hankering towards a series of smoker stands my father owned. Every few years he'd oust the old one and replace it with a more up-to-date model. The style and shape of these stands were ideal for my purposes. The first one I ever took to was made of carved wood, thicker at the bottom end, with a table like a circular skirt around the elaborately carved central column. The thick end provided a good basis for necessary friction of movement when I placed the stand between my legs. Later, I fancied an aluminium version, 1950s styling, with two swinging tables that rotated around a slim length of tubing on top of which was an ashtray and matchbox holder. At the bottom of this slim tube was a raised section that flattened down to the floor in a series of circular ridges. At the point where the tubing met the base I positioned my crotch, and with both arms extended up to grasp the swinging tables I was set for a jolly good time while lying on the floor.

There was a risk of discovery in this practice, and while it might be suggested that this added excitement to my enjoyment I know that I was much too scared of my father's brutality to feel anything like that. It may have been a silent act of rebellion, but if that is true then it bypassed my conscious awareness, and I always chose my moments carefully. Afternoons, after school, my young brother played in the street; my mum worked as a school cleaner which meant she arrived home much later; my father was a wharf-labourer and my sister had to travel to school some distance away. In other years my mother ran a boarding house so although opportunity could not be counted on as a daily occurrence, it was still possible to find an odd hour here and there. I think the strongest pull towards using these cigarette stands, and in later years other items, the handle end of a hairbrush for example, was because I had absorbed some negativity about the female body. It was faulty though, not strong enough to influence me greatly.

Brought up in the 1940s/1950s, I'd been taught by my mother that the word for 'down there' was *shame*, what I did in the toilet was called *wee-wee* if it was liquid and yellow and *pain* if it was hard and brown. My mother, like many others, had an attitude that reflected gloom and doom.

Mothers did change their attitudes when daughters grew older, became adults, such adulthood signified not by age but by events like marriage and/or childbirth. Then daughters would find themselves admitted to the world of secrets. Initiation over, recognition could be gained of the inconvenience and pressure, the expectations placed on women's lives. But if a girl knew this too soon? Well, that was an open invitation for the worst of disasters to fall upon her. Ignorance, avoidance of any questions or discussion, passing on the barest information and often misinformation, was the order of the day, intended to protect and curb maybe, yet it could generate curiosity in the young.

I grew up avoiding any contact with my body. My hands never stroked or caressed those bits of me that might have been aroused by such contact. I was cut off from this sort of pleasure and can only describe a stark need from that place between my legs that I would not have been able to find with my hands, but oh, how well it responded when something firm and hard was placed near it. The habit was formed, the die was cast. Sexual excitement and pleasure do not always conform to intellectual arguments. Rare are the times even now when I use my fingers to encourage an orgasm during those moments of private pleasure.

Since the mid 1970s a lot has been said about female sexuality. Sometimes, I've felt coerced to fall in with a line of thought that made me feel wrong and distanced from my own experience. I prefer now to think that what has happened to me cannot be ignored. I find that I am content to live with the choice my earlier self made, and no, I don't have a collection of smoker stands, but I have owned a series of vibrators. There have been women who've challenged me for using a vibrator, suggested that I will never love myself until I can arouse full orgasmic delight by using my own fingers on my clitoris. I've opted for my own definition of sexuality rather than subscribe to someone else's view.

There were distinct advantages for me in the practice of masturbation in childhood and well beyond. I think of it as an act of love between me and myself. For as long as I can remember I've always talked to myself, and in a way, felt that there were two of me (I may be schizophrenic but I'll always have each other), for there have been, and still are, arguments I have with myself. I accept this now in understanding that I am a complex person. The atmosphere at home was charged with hostility and fear and we children were caught in the crossfire of our parent's marital conflicts and frustrations that could flare into violence as quickly as a struck match can produce flame.

I think my physical need was a way of giving myself something. Comfort? Love? It doesn't matter what I'd call it, the important thing is that it was intuitive. I responded to that and am still learning about the ways it works positively for me. I didn't think about what I was doing and so avoided any internal wrangling. Perhaps for this reason, continuity was assured.

Masturbation made it possible for me to circumvent some of the destruction that threatened to make inroads on my sexual identity via the physical and sexual abuse I received from my father. His hands on my body made me shudder with nauseous revulsion. I had a history of masturbation long before the rape that took place the year I was twelve. That small history proved surprisingly resistant to feelings of shame and blame, though I would not wish to deny the complexity, confusion, anger and pain I had to work through in coming to terms with my father's power over me. What I'm saying is that there was less damage done to my sexuality than might be expected. I was helped in this process by long-held feelings of hatred and contempt for that man, my father. Hating him meant there was no room for ambivalence, no compassion for him in later years. He was violent, selfish and cruel. In short, he was a bully. The only act of kindness I can ever recall from him happened one night towards the end of World War Two. He brought home some threepenny chocolates and handed them around to us kids. It's the only positive memory of him I have, and all I can say is that it was not enough. It never will be.

He died when I was forty-three and living on the west coast of England. I wasn't told of his death until nine months later. I was furious. Now I would never know whether or not I'd have chosen to go to his funeral. I'd often wished for his death as a child, willing it on him while silently standing before him, meek and obedient. But behind those eyes that dropped before his gaze I lived with a passion and verve he never saw. It's been a long time since I felt the hatred; that died out long ago. It takes energy to hate someone, and usually means the connection is still strong. I withdrew the energy but maintain my opinion. It took me a long while to realize how complex other women's healing processes are after childhood rape, while mine seems so single-minded by comparison. My father was what he was and I accept no responsibility for him or for his actions. Eliminating the effects of his power has been very hard but I was always determined and feel strongly that masturbation acted as a core of inner self, to protect me from any long-term injury to my sexuality.

But if I describe my sexuality as an area protected intuitively by masturbation, the same cannot be said for how I feel about closeness and being touched by others. There was no affection in our family and my mother gave me to understand quite early on that even to kiss someone was to spread germs. Added to that was the real isolation of growing up in a household where violence was the norm. I sought retreat somewhere deep inside me and touch was part of the noise and fuss that heralded an assault on the outer walls of my being. I avoided any gesture of warmth from teachers and adults, put my faith in the comfort of words and learned too well when I'd been beaten or hurt to talk to myself about such pain. It became difficult to allow someone close, other than for the sexual act. Only in the last few years have I managed to gain some resolution about this via the support and caring persistence of my lover.

It was to be a contradiction played out through many years and with little insight until after my marriage ended. My distrust of men was at odds with the conditioning that said marriage and children were a woman's destiny. I didn't know how to side-step this conditioning and at the age of thirteen made a bargain with God that I'd be good, would suffer through what was left of my childhood years, so long as he gave me three little girls whom I could mother and love and make up to as some sort of substitution for myself. There was no man in my fantasies, for the focus was clearly on having children, and I had a need so urgent to have children of my own that I accepted the conditioned message and looked at the men I dated as though mentally auditioning them for the role of husband and father. Having sons in the 1960s seemed a cruel joke. But I chose to be a different kind of parent and this has given me hope, pleasure and fun in being the mother of sons.

I have masturbation to thank for getting me through the 1950s unscathed. My older sister married when I was sixteen. I didn't like watching her life change so abruptly with marriage and then motherhood. I made myself a promise that same year. I'd not think about marriage until I was twenty-one, nor would I allow myself to be talked into a sexual relationship.

My teen years were marked by poverty and I wanted something more in that distant future. I had a low-paid job in a chemist's shop and lived in a bed and breakfast house on a sparse diet of peanut butter sandwiches, toast, baked beans and cheap bars of chocolate. I reasoned that a girl's virginity was all she had to bargain with out there in that scary world and I wasn't going to sell myself short. Morality was intertwined with my reasoning, and while my mother had expounded the view that cleanliness was nearer to godliness I privately thought that virginity held until marriage would ensure me a better chance for a brighter future here on earth.

My background, my schooling in a convent run by an order of Irish nuns, my job, my friends, provided no opportunity to connect me with my lesbianism nor did I glimpse any instances of such a lifestyle that might have provided food for thought. I doubt that I'd have paid much attention though, for marriage in Australia in the late 1950s was like the Italian liners so many people travelled overseas on, usually after months or years working two jobs and saving hard. It cost me too much to live from week to week to consider such a trip, but with the help of Hollywood movies and books I could daydream about marriage as a wonderful voyage to another way of life and save myself up for that. One day it would happen to me and I'd be prepared. It wasn't so much a decision about whether or not to marry, no, the emphasis was on *when*. The alternative had already been labelled 'left on the shelf'. Little wonder so many of us thought in terms of assets and trade. It clearly was a market, the marriage market.

My friends and I went to dances where we met boys and, sooner or later, married the one who stuck around. We were still going to those dances when late-night closing began in pubs. The transition between dance halls and fancy pubs with miniature dance floors was easy to make. Being escorted home by a drunk or less-than-sober fellow with amorous inclinations required tact and a few evasive strategies. Masturbation provided me with an autonomy that did little to diminish my growing curiosity but that assisted greatly in allowing common sense to prevail. If I got stirred up while petting with a boy in his car then you can bet I was frantic and eager by the time I got inside. What he did about his arousal was his problem, I was taking care of mine.

I understood that there were forces at work in my own body that might lead me into a disastrous marriage (or worse) following a night of frolic with a man who'd use wonderfully romantic words and not mean them the minute the sperm left his penis. I was unmoved by arguments from boys that I didn't trust them, had 'led them on' and was a cock-teaser. I already knew how much I took responsibility for my sexual feelings and had no hesitation in sarcastically suggesting that their problem was not my problem. Such an outspoken viewpoint did not mix well with long-term bonds, so although there were a number of boys I went out with there were only two that I ever 'went steady' with and I later married one of them. I had strict rules for where I could be touched (above the waist only, though this changed with the two men I trusted) and I held myself solely responsible for what happened. I felt that only I could be relied on to get myself through to a time when I hoped to be better able to handle close physical contact.

So far, my whole life had been based on reaction. Reaction to the violent home of my childhood, reaction from the poverty, the hardships, the day-to-day grind. I hungered for something different and sought acceptance from a world I'd glimpsed from where I stood, on the wrong side of the tracks. I wanted respectability more than anything else. Respectability would be like an umbrella I could stand under, my future husband would hold it aloft, providing protection from my parents and the past. It was a man's umbrella, large and serviceable. Excitement? Ah well, I could provide that and a whole number of other things too, but he, and only he, could provide that umbrella of respectability. I yearned for the opportunity to do the job better than my parents ever had, to prove something, to myself more than others. I felt children had a right to be wanted. I hadn't been. I'd make sure my children were, moving heaven and earth to bring about the best possible circumstances for their security, starting before they were born.

The two men I did trust had one thing in common. Neither of them pressed me to be sexual. We kissed, we petted, we created an atmosphere of intimacy but such closeness did not threaten me and I realize now how surface-based it was when compared to the lesbian relationships I've had since. When I married I had definite goals, saving for a house and waiting to have children until a greater sense of financial security could be achieved. I would still have been a virgin when I married at almost twenty-three had it not been that I grew a little rebellious four nights before the wedding. I drank a lot of cheap wine and we went back to the flat, I invited him in for the usual cup of tea and a cuddle, and got on with the job of changing my virginal state. The agony of this experience could have triggered, but didn't, a memory of the much earlier rape which I had blocked out of my mind almost as soon as it happened. Thinking the pain and discomfort was normal, I suffered for four long weeks. The distress was intensified each time I passed urine. When finally I was sent to a specialist, he insisted that my new husband refrain from seeking what the specialist called 'his conjugal rights' while I underwent a three-month period of healing treatment.

When my first son was born we moved to the suburbs – not the middle-class suburbs where prosperity flourished with two-car garages and split-level living was spacious and elegant and wives played tennis while the children were at school and husbands earned salaries that were paid directly into a bank account. No, our house was in the western suburbs, made of cheap fibro that could be replaced panel by panel if the kids were too rough with a cricket ball or the removalists were careless with your furniture. Designed as a rectangle, squat beneath the inevitable red roof, our new abode was small. The down deposit had been low, the weekly mortgage payments a struggle at first and we agreed I'd have to work for at least eighteen months to pay the second mortgage which amounted to £150. My husband's wage was so small we'd had to ask his boss to write a letter to the building society that said he earned more than he did. But still the house was ours with its three bedrooms, open-plan living room cum kitchen cum dining room, bathroom, outside laundry and a yard big enough for children to play. The ground was thick mud and I sank to my knees the first time I hung clothes on the rotary clothes line.

The first three years of that marriage were good. We moved into the house during the second year and our first son was born a week before our third anniversary. I'd given up work only six weeks before the birth. Two years later came the second son and six months after that I was referred to a psychiatrist, immersed in depression and classified within weeks as a paranoid schizophrenic. What had gone wrong? Masturbation was no help now, that was for sure. I didn't even want to think about things like that. All I wanted to do was sleep.

The culmination of things unresolved from the past, the dissatisfactions of the present, and the reality of being denied daughters while finding myself the mother of two sons, meant I reeled under the weight of irrational feelings. I did not reject my children or withhold love and attention from them, but I did have unrealistic expectations of my ability to manage while dealing with an unfocused but nonetheless real agony of disappointment.

I'd also hoped to have a better life than my mother, more money for example, and could not yet face the recognition that my choices had not provided me with the safety I'd sought. My husband was a familiar stranger, rooted to routine and unwilling to move beyond the roles we'd assumed since I'd given up work. I was locked in and locked out. Locked into a non-negotiable marriage and locked out of the expectations of love and family that I'd longed for with the hungry need of an orphan child.

The depression lasted with great severity for three years. We were both confused and beaten by it. The main difference between us was that while I writhed and struggled to break free and desperately sought some dialogue between us, he fended me off with excuses that hid his fear, with platitudes and clichés about 'men as breadwinners and women as homemakers'. He wanted a quiet life, supper on the table at six o'clock, a wife who darned socks, ironed clothes and listened more than talked. Why couldn't I be like that, he wanted to know? If he was thoughtless or hurtful he expected to be able to say sorry and forget all about it until the next time. When we went anywhere together he had to be the one who sat behind the wheel of the car, had to drink as much as our male friends, had to have separate pocket money. Things were just like that, women didn't need these things, why didn't I understand that? I became so angry that at times it seemed like a perpetual state. He labelled me 'a bitch'. I remembered my mother's sharp tongue. Now I understood a little better why she used it so much. Unable to compete with my bitter accusations my husband began to use his fists. That was the end for me. Almost thirteen years to the day had passed since we'd got married. It was time to call it quits. He moved back with his mother, I breathed a sigh of relief and stretched myself to keep up with the demands of children and home as well as the job I'd had for some time.

During the years of my marriage my sexual responses to my husband had varied from excitement and interest to lack of enthusiasm, boredom, and finally a revulsion if he even came close. I took up masturbation again with vigour now, understanding more about what it meant. I bought my first vibrator and conducted a lengthy conversation with a young woman in a department store about the merits of this one or that. She believed me when I said I needed it to massage my neck and while she expounded the advantages of one brand over another I was evaluating the shape and imagining how well they'd nestle against that lower part of my anatomy. I went through months of experimentation, learning to caress and fondle myself but feeling self-conscious and reluctant at times. Passages in books became triggers for lusty feelings and I began to understand that I was 'turned on' more by words than by anything visual. It was a time of learning. I gave the kids the biggest bedroom, made another bedroom into a playroom for them and placing a three-foot mattress on the floor in the third room, set up the space in readiness for a life of my own. I didn't for one moment consider that I'd ever have a sexual relationship again, believing firmly that if it hadn't worked out with one man, it was unlikely I'd be able to go down the same road with another.

Sexual fantasies about women came even before I began attending the meetings at the women's health centre. I was embarrassed but made no serious attempt to stop the fantasies. In them, although I played the initiating role, I did not know what to do after I'd mentally touched a woman's body, enjoying the idea of foreplay, then ... nothing. I did not know how to proceed beyond that. During those first visits to the health centre I was wary, having been told that sometimes lesbians went to these meetings. I wore a jacket with a fake fur collar, deciding that this would show what side of the fence I was on. I'd never liked the jacket, given as a gift by my husband the previous Mother's Day, but I wore it now, believing I was making a clear statement. After the third meeting I hung the jacket at the back of the wardrobe and never wore it again.

I took to wearing ties. I found a couple in one of the bedroom drawers my husband had used. I liked the white one with my navy shirt and pants, the red one I wore with a grey school shirt my older brother had given me years before. One of the women joked with me about these ties. I told her I was wearing them to create a different style of dress. She thought otherwise and said so. I wasn't shocked as I listened to what she had to say but my legs shook when I got up to go home. She phoned that weekend, invited me to her house. I'd found two sisters, twins who lived nearby, who agreed to come babysit for me. They'd stay overnight and I'd leave a supply of small treats in the fridge as well as giving each of them a bit of pocket money, which meant I had some time away from the children. I went willingly the next week to the woman's house. I knew what was happening and my nervousness was not because I was reluctant but because I felt awe-struck by the dramatic changes taking place within me. It's hard to explain the nature of my relationship with that woman or even to question now if there was any alternative. She was married, had been for many, many years. She'd chosen marriage even though she knew how strongly attracted she was to women. She explained that as a girl she could see ahead only a life of isolation and misery and, scared of that, she'd made a choice that all in all she did not regret.

I'd been separated from my husband for a year and the funny thing was that a few weeks after beginning this new relationship I went back to my marriage. To this day, I am not absolutely clear about the reasons why. Was I scared or still trapped? I was in the same small house we'd bought many years before. It wasn't much of a house and the size meant there was little chance of overstuffing it with furniture. We'd decorated it with cheap brown carpet, plastic light fittings, embossed silver wallpaper with large circles set in triangles in a continuous pattern that I'd once thought modern and in the best taste but about which I now felt a tinge of embarrassment when my new women friends came for tea. It was a house I'd created, my children were growing up there, I felt an obligation to them to stay put. Such things are not easily dislodged, no matter how stirring and profound the changes going on beneath the surface. He came back but I was a different person. He said he was too but the months proved him wrong.

I fought now with a greater articulation and understanding of the issues involved. I told him about the new relationship and put it to him that he did not have to accept it but that if he wanted to come back then he'd have to understand that I viewed it 'as an extension of friendship'. He said he could cope, didn't mind so long as I was discreet; indeed he remarked he'd noted my attraction to women a long time ago and well, it was something I'd have to get out of my system. I refused to surrender my new-found independence or play any role I saw as unequal. I fought him uncompromisingly and no longer doled out compassion for his apologies after the event. I wanted more freedom. I wanted respect. I was willing to give these things but I had to have them too. When it became abundantly clear that he was unwilling to make genuine changes I withdrew from any further negotiations with him but did not make this apparent until there was nothing left to hold me.

When I walked away, the second time at the end of two years, I found I'd expelled any remaining doubts I might have had about marriage, male conditioning and life in the suburbs. He wouldn't leave so I did, taking the boys with me. These days when women tell me how they yearn for a revolution I tell them to look around, to take note of the vast number of women who are walking away from stale and unsatisfactory marriages. I think it is a revolution and should be seen as such. When I remember the situations my mother and her sisters lived with, year in, year out, I know that the daughters of that generation often use the knowledge gained to reach out for something more, something better, and I'm one of them.

I had kept in touch with my woman lover though our times together were few. I felt grateful to her for giving me essential knowledge about myself but now I had to accept that she was still living with her choices and I was about to explore a broader horizon for mine. I ended the relationship but affirmed that we would go on being friends, good friends. I told her my plans and she listened and we talked and then I left. I could at last say the word 'lesbian' and not shrink away from the implications involved. The time for doubt, the time for guilt, had now passed.

I'd masturbated through that last two-year period of my marriage, preferring to seek comfort and pleasure with myself during those times when contact with my husband was at a low ebb or in a state of crisis. I can understand how my lesbianism fits comfortably with the autonomy masturbation provided. Being a lesbian means a number of things to me but most importantly it means that I am attracted to women sexually and emotionally and have no hesitation in accepting this and all it implies about me. I understand that I have always been strong, independent, unable to 'buckle under to any man' throughout my life. The complaints that used to be made about my stubbornness, my strong will and forthright manner made it difficult for me to feel free of men's judgments. Strength does not mean I carry great weights or am able to thump a bloke in a pub if he's rude. It does mean that I have an ability to see myself through things, that I try to be clear about the support I can give to others and that I'm unstinting about following through with what I've said I'll do, as lover, friend, colleague, co-worker, activist.

There are still men in my life besides my two sons who are both in their twenties. These men are friends I care about and they have added to my understanding about childhood years. By their willingness to acknowledge the vulnerabilities within themselves, they have permitted me to feel eased in areas where my spirit had been left feeling bloodied and raw. As a young wife I was willing to accept society's roles for men and women so long as he did his bit and lived up to the image that was supposed to protect as well as provide. But my life wasn't like that. I learned to doubt his willingness to see things through, to listen, to give comfort, in short, to 'be there' at all. I handled everything from bank statements and bills to funeral arrangements, hospital admissions, holiday plans and, eventually, the sale of the house. Female relatives had often joked, advising that I should let him think he'd thought of a plan or won the argument, but this I decided was dishonest. What man could possibly want a women to protect his ego to that extent? What man could possibly have such a frail ego? Too many I discovered. Far too many.

This inherent capacity and need for autonomy, whether it be called strong, independent, whatever, has its roots in my habit of masturbation. Like I said in the beginning, it is as familiar to me as washing my hair or making a bed. I am far more experimental with it now and not as secretive about it as I used to be. I can talk about it openly with the woman who shares my life.

When first I began to write for this book I felt exposed and concerned about how my words might be interpreted. I've moved past those feelings in part though it would be foolish to say I've left them behind. I've not ever found any books that spoke to me of my experience and there has not been enough discussion on the subject for me to know if there are other women who have used it as I have or have had similar childhood experiences. The urge to name and define, to give voice to an aspect of female experience, is still uppermost in my mind. I like to think I can trust my intuition, trust it and heed it and learn. That intuition is a genuine link with that small child within me, and although I'm past the half-century mark it becomes stronger as I continue to explore the landscape of my childhood.

I'm saving up to leave my husband
Kate Ashcroft

'I'm saving up to leave my husband.' So goes the first line of a recent poem of mine. It wasn't until I talked it through with several friends that I realized reaching this point has been a thirty-year process. Part of that process was working through my own attitudes to my sex and sexuality.

The question I ask is, how did I get from hopeful romantic teenager to middle-aged celibate with an acquired dislike of anything relating to the vagina? This is a painful journey and not unique to me. Every woman has some portion of my experience. The wonderful thing is we all handle situations differently and the results need not be disastrous.

My first boyfriend entered my life on my sixteenth birthday. My mother and father were loving, trusting people and I had been well indoctrinated in the belief that 'good girls don't'. I spent the next two years holding him off although I often felt the urge to give in. Losing my virginity was traumatic mainly because it wasn't the result of a mutually arrived at moment of passion, but of his not being prepared to wait any longer. His forcing, although not brutal, was painful and left me feeling that sex was something for men to enjoy, women to endure. I did change my mind in the summer prior to my eighteenth birthday.

His parents were away, the weather was warm, the moment romantic. This time no forcing, but a mutually enjoyable sexual experience and my first orgasm. Unfortunately it resulted in a pregnancy that would colour the rest of my life. 'Good girls don't.' I had, and it soon became obvious that I had. While my parents and family didn't judge me, offering me support and love instead, my erstwhile boyfriend did. Before the words 'It's a girl' could touch his ears he had left the city for pastures new. Despite the upset of the moment

I heaved a sigh of relief. I had come to realize that we would never have made it work. He, I found out later, had a girl in every parish and was escaping not one unwanted pregnancy but three.

I never considered anything other than keeping my baby. My parents would provide back-up and I would work, the only problem being how I would be accepted by my peer group once I returned to work. A new job seemed the answer, somewhere where I was unknown and could make new friendships. It had long been my practice not to socialize with friends at work, so it wasn't difficult to live two different lives. After my third interview I decided not to admit to being an unmarried mother. Each time I was honest with my potential employer he suddenly found a good reason to turn me down. My fourth application proved successful, as I had told personnel I had been off work for four months looking after my sick mother. Like all lies, this lie once uttered had to continue and caused me many moments of deep guilt.

Being single and seemingly unburdened with husband or children proved difficult. Peer-group pressure demanded I join in, accept the invites to nights out, parties, etc. I endeavoured to keep this to a minimum. My parents weren't the stumbling block; they were only too glad to care for my daughter and allow me a social life. It was my deceit that bothered me. I couldn't cope with the thought of meeting a boy known to my working friends and having to lie my way through and beyond the first evening. This was the most difficult period you can imagine. Honesty had always been a byword for me, so the stress became almost unbearable. All the conversations in and out of work were based on who was getting engaged to whom. Weddings were being planned, it seemed, by the minute. I began to feel I was some sort of cuckoo in the singles' nest.

My problem resolved itself, in a sense. I met somebody I liked. Saturday nights were always reserved for going out for a drink with my parents, just the local, just for an hour. There he was across the pub, someone I liked the look of, someone who, if I read the body language correctly, was interested in me. Over the weeks we nodded, then said hello, and finally got close enough to exchange information, pleasantries, an invitation out and an acceptance.

This time honesty would serve me as it had in the past. I resolved not to lie. On the second date I took a deep breath and poured out my 'sin'. I think he was shocked, but willing to listen and give me a chance to say all I had to say. Our 'romance' developed very quickly, but sex was out of the question. This was my decision. Naturally I was afraid of lightning striking twice.

A strange twist of fate occurred after we'd been going together for about five weeks. I noticed he started to bring up the subject of my baby rather a lot. Maybe he was having second thoughts? I couldn't face a protracted discussion on the subject so I wrote him a letter, basically saying I felt he should seriously consider his position and his feelings about me. I gave him two weeks to think it over, giving him a date and time to call on me if he decided to continue the relationship, but saying I would understand if he chose not to. I thought all I had to do was sit it out for a fortnight. If he didn't turn up I could feel sorry for myself for a while and then get on with my life.

Four days before the deadline my father died suddenly. My brother, not thinking to ask me, called on my boyfriend at work to tell him the news and, without realizing it, used the emotional push of telling him I was in a very distressed condition and desperately needed his support and love. He worded this appeal as if I had sent the message. My brother always was convinced women couldn't survive without men to prop them up. I was unaware of what had happened until long afterwards. I simply accepted the excuse that my boyfriend had made his decision earlier than the set date and felt grateful I didn't have to cope with losing him on top of losing the most caring, understanding father anyone ever had.

Due to this fluke I built up a great feeling of gratitude towards my (then) future husband. I was going to achieve the thing I wanted most of all – respectability. I still didn't realize how much the opinions, hopes and dreams of my female friends had rubbed off on me. If my father had lived I know he would have discussed the situation with me. His wisdom, while I'd often bucked against it, had been infallible. He wasn't there, and my mother could not help. She was suddenly bereaved, so there was nothing in life she could concentrate on except her loss.

The relationship moved on until we reached the point at which I felt comfortable with suggesting that we might see how sexually compatible we were. I expected so much. Here was a gentle, sexually unaware man whom I felt I really loved. This would be wonderful, I told myself. It turned out to be a non-event. I realized he was inexperienced and might need some time. Even then I felt there was something that was causing him to hold something of himself back. I should have questioned him then. I never did, my fault I know, but by then I was in love with the idea of marriage. I suppose I didn't want to dig too deeply.

On my wedding day the trigger that released something of the real person in him was a large quantity of drink. I found myself facing a man I really didn't know. I was suddenly 'no good', a 'slag', and he told me he wanted to hear all over again all the details of my previous relationship. The cross-examination continued into the early evening until drink finally took the rest of its toll and silence followed.

My expectations (sexual, that is) never flagged. I truly believed things would improve. As I had become pregnant again immediately I married, life took over from experimentation. Sex had to take something of a back seat. All the usual things filled my life — planning for another baby while building up a comfortable home, worrying about bills, coping day to day. Whenever I tried to broach the subject of sex my husband became embarrassed. I echoed his embarrassment, and nothing was resolved.

It wasn't that he didn't have a good sex drive. He insisted on sex every night, but I soon realized that was all it was — 'sex'. I wasn't even certain that he enjoyed it. I felt I couldn't really ask. I often lay awake afterwards wondering what was going through his mind. My third child was born just a year after the second. No time to wish or wonder, only time to cope yet again.

He started to drink heavily after my third child was born. Every night 9.30 found him putting his coat on to return at 10.45 a little the worse for wear. I was expected to have the house neatly tidied, dishes wished, nightie on and be in a suitable frame of mind for bed.

I think it was about this time that I started to 'fake it'. I reasoned that if he felt more 'accomplished' sexually he might respect himself more, and it might therefore follow he would start to talk to me about sexual matters. I led myself to believe I could achieve some level of understanding via this method. It never happened, of course. His disappointment was too deeply rooted. I suppose he felt cheated because life had made decisions for him. I could never understand why he said he loved me yet still felt the need to drink in order to have sex with me. I started to believe it was something to do with how I looked, that the shortcomings were all mine.

Somebody asked me recently if I'd indulged in sexual fantasies at that time. I said I hadn't, but on reflection I suppose I had. I was working as a cashier in a large factory. It was mainly male workers who used the canteen in which I worked. Some of them were friendly to the point of having to be put in their place. At least one or two in the three years I worked there caught my eye. I never did anything about it, because whenever my fantasy reached the stage of undressing in front of them, I imagined myself dying of shame. However, I recall using an imagined romantic/sexy situation with the current heart-throb to arouse myself to warm responsiveness while in bed with my husband. It appeared that the more aroused I became the less my husband liked it, so I stopped that line of attack and sank back into sexual boredom.

Over the years my acting talents took over from any real sexual urges I may have had. I would find myself looking at the wart on his chin and working through all sorts of things in my head. It really became an 'out of body experience', a long sexual yawn.

Eventually I 'settled' for what I had and suppressed the need for anything more. I feel I could have continued in this vein forever if it had not been for a change in my husband's attitude. Some years ago, I'm not sure exactly when, the accusations started. You know that moment, pre-sex, when maybe you talk a little, get the thoughts of the day out of the way and so go on to foreplay? For us it became the time when he would name men I had had affairs with. Needless to say, I had never had sex with anyone but him since our marriage. But he would become so verbally aggressive it was terrifying. These accusations built up over the years to intolerable levels. I know it was during this period I really 'turned off' sexually.

I still acted the part to keep the peace, but any feelings I may have had were very quickly dying. Every form of emotional bullying known to humankind he used. I coped because I challenged each changing mood, each threat as it presented itself. There was a moment finally when I realized he was using repeated methods to scare me, or bring me to tears. Then I knew I was on top of it. He was running out of effective methods of punishment.

What I really wanted was to understand why every moment of our lives was filled with anger. There were times when I felt my husband wanted this knowledge too, but his apologies and tears were always followed by long silences, and bouts of uncontrolled rage, directed at me.

Eventually I decided to use my energies *for* myself rather than in defence of myself. As the family was grown and I faced the prospect of middle age locked in the same situation, I knew a change was needed.

Returning to education sounds like a phrase from a pamphlet on 'things to do with a boring life'. It wasn't like that. I hoped a new interest for me might rub off on my relationship. I might be able to inject something external, even get my husband interested in something outside his obsession with my non-existent infidelities. Of course it didn't work. How foolish I was to imagine it could. All my new life gave to him was heightened insecurity. He saw it as my having even more opportunity to meet other men, have even more affairs.

I suppose it was, but I didn't. I didn't because by this time I felt so awful about my body, so insecure about my ability to 'do it' – after all, I don't seem ever to have satisfied my husband, so maybe I'm no good at it, was my attitude. I never wanted to be tested sexually again. I dreaded (and I use that word in its fullest sense) anyone making a pass. I couldn't cope with even the slightest sexual innuendo. All my years of maturing, all my kids, all the sexual moments in my life were no longer worth anything. I felt like a shy, sexually unaware teenager in the company of sexually active adults. I have always been a 'blusher', but it got worse, and I avoided 'adult' conversations whenever I could.

This situation didn't alter very much until about two years ago. I know I still had some sex drive because I could still fantasize about the odd individual who visually turned me on.

Tom Selick was one such beauty, but most of that was TV packaging, I suppose. Then the menopause which had been lurking without being a problem for several years hit me with all its force. I lost my sex drive. Nothing moved me at all. Everything was a turn off, rather than a turn on. The good thing about it was that I couldn't even act any more. This baffled me totally. I'd believed you could always 'fake it', but no, I really couldn't. I lay impassive, almost comatose, during the sex act. It became immediately obvious to my husband that something different was happening. We didn't discuss it in depth as I would have liked, but we talked a little more than we ever had on the subject. I told him I wished to move into my own room and that I really didn't ever want sex again.

Looking back on the last two years I honestly think he breathed a sigh of relief. All sorts of questions go through my head, the main one being could he have struggled through his whole life without a real knowledge or understanding of his own sexuality? I remember a particularly bad period about ten years ago when he was convinced everyone was talking about him, saying he was a homosexual. I couldn't understand it at the time, but felt all I could do was reassure him he wasn't and that people certainly were not saying such things. I wonder if that false situation of our coming together after the death of my father didn't force both of us into accepting the so-called 'norm' of marriage? Maybe we both needed more time to find ourselves and recognize fully our sexual needs?

I have to remember he was a virgin. How could he possibly have known what was best for himself? I on the other hand had had only one previous relationship. Our mutual yet separate celibacy has not, I should say, resolved all the problems. But it has got rid of some of the underlying anger that I could see bubbling inside my husband for so many years and it has given me space and time to think about my own needs. After a lifetime of 'making allowances' my celibacy has given me time to peel back the layers, see the mistakes, recognize my own confusion and my husband's inability to voice his needs and fears. I feel I suckled and protected the man until my own identity was almost overwhelmed, but that my protectiveness did him no real service. It gave him something to hide behind, fuelled his uncertainty and left us both empty.

Over the last two years I have been very aware of the support and help of other women. Family and good friends have all contributed to my 'seeing' myself again. This is especially true of my eldest daughter who returned to live near me with my two grandchildren two years ago. She had divorced her husband and was set to make her own life, returning to the independent girl and woman I had always known. She told me soon after her arrival in the city, 'Mum, I'm a lesbian.' She talked about her sexuality so easily, took such joy in her self-knowledge. I breathed a sigh of relief and thought thank goodness she at least knows where she's at – I'm still trying to find the map.

I think I feel the stirrings of a sex drive returning. Someone told me that it might. I've discovered that masturbation is great. I giggle at the thought that I get more out of my own tentative experiments than from thirty years of marriage. I've started to wonder if there is anything to be afraid of in extra-marital relations, and I don't feel guilty at the thought. I believe there's hope for me yet. I'm still not sure about my sexuality. I have to be honest, and I believe I have a lot of self-examination ahead of me. What I am not doing is shutting any doors. Yes, I am still saving up to leave my husband. I feel he may cope much better without me, and why should I cramp his style?

Social security was the best husband I ever had
Kate

I was brought up in the north-west of England in the 1930s, a black child born of an African father and a white, English mother. My father was a staunch Roman Catholic, my mother was Church of England.

My father had come to England as a young boy, working his passage by sea. He used to tell me how he'd been looked after by 'old-timers', men who had come over here in Queen Victoria's time. My father could neither read nor write, but he knew a great deal about African history (it is a eurocentric view that people who can't read or write are ignorant) and had a strong sense of the oral history which is very much a part of African culture. There was a feeling of pride handed down to me from my father and I've carried that pride with me through the years.

Lots of black people used to meet in our house during the 1940s and 1950s – political activists who were coming across to negotiate freedom from colonialism and independence for Africa – and I remember meeting Kenyatta and Nkrumah. I was brought up in an atmosphere of political struggle against imperialism, though my father would not have been able to describe it in that way.

My mother was very bright but lacked formal education. Her family – originally Durham miners – rejected her for marrying a black man. My father was considerably taller than the British working class of that time and my mother used to want to show us kids off as we were all big and strapping. We were the new blood from Africa, she would say, putting some goodness into the family.

Employment was a key issue for my parents throughout their lives and my father was always seeking ways and means of earning money to provide for us. Mother had a number of jobs; she was a tailoress. In those days, before World War Two, few black people, male or female, had steady work. Black men could sometimes get jobs as seamen, but were expected to bribe the supervisor for the privilege.

As a white woman married to a black man, my mother was often more active and visible than her husband. For example, it was my mother who found us our first house when we moved from the city to a large coastal town, but when she produced a black husband and black children the white residents started a petition, ours being the first black family to move there. My mother always defended us, but I know that for her racism was secondary, not primary. I'm sure she used to feel it, but she didn't feel it as we did. She couldn't.

I feel strongly that the discrimination I've experienced has come because of my blackness rather than because I am a woman. I think it's important to remember that black women and black men served the same function – we both suffered the lash, and being women didn't save us. While white women were mothers, black women were known as breeders. For me, then, sexism is there, but first of all comes the reality that I am black. First I am a black person; second I am a woman.

I find it hard to say who I was close to as a small child; I was something of a loner. I used to sit beneath my bed or in a tree trunk, thinking and thinking. Like most black children at that time, I could daydream myself into white aspirations.

My father used to tell me about black women in America who straightened their hair, and I would say how awful that was, to want straight hair, yet I would be in my bedroom playing around with a scarf over my hair almost every day. Sometimes white people would call me Topsy, like the book, and I would feel resentful. I was always being asked if I was black all over. I used to look out for black women to identify with – I thought Carmen Miranda was black, and how wonderful she was and that I was like her. When I was sixteen my closest role model was my Auntie Alma, who played in *Showboat* with Paul Robeson.

I was seven when I started junior school and it is from this year that I can clearly pinpoint changes in the way I was treated. Questions were asked that I didn't know how to answer — questions about why we'd moved. There was always the assumption that we'd come from a city slum, though nothing could have been further from the truth.

I remember going to a Christmas party and winning a doll — at least I was told I'd won it, but there followed some discussion among a group of adults and in the end I was given another present, an artificial Christmas tree. Another ticket was drawn in order that a white child could be given that beautifully dressed, blond-haired doll. If I'd been asked to say what those adults had been thinking, I would have bet they believed that doll was too bloody good to give a black kid. But my mother was so pleased with the tree, and by then I'd become so used to the way white people could treat me, it didn't seem appropriate to tell my parents. Many black children don't tell their parents all the hurtful things they encounter in and out of school; only when it gets too much to bear do they divulge to an adult what has happened to them.

That occasion was such an overt incident of racism I could not hide the knowledge from myself in later incidents. White people would often stroke my hair, 'a touch for luck' they would say. Two weeks back an elderly white woman, a neighbour, reached out to touch my hair. I was furious. 'Don't touch my fucking hair,' I yelled. It brought back all the resentment I'd felt as a child.

Although we were a big family and we talked about lots of things at home, sex was never discussed. My periods began the year I was eleven, which was also the year I sat for the scholarship exam, later replaced by the eleven-plus. My mother explained that this bleeding would happen every month but that I must not in any circumstances 'let a lad near me'. I didn't understand what she meant and felt very scared. I also took in a message of somehow being unclean. As an older woman I've learned about some religious attitudes to women's bleeding times and I can remember my father distancing himself from us in similar ways. I stopped going swimming after that. There were parts of my body that were darker than others and I became overly conscious of how I looked. It seems to me now that having begun menstruation my parents closed the bedroom door and that was the end of that. When my daughter was growing up I remembered my younger self and was probably more help to her because of that experience.

After the scholarship exam I was very excited. I'd been told I'd passed. I waited for the post each day throughout the weeks after school broke up. By the end of August, with still no word, my father told my mother to go and see the people at the education department. She came home that afternoon with very red-looking eyes. Yes, she'd been told, I had won a scholarship, but they'd allocated the place to another child because they'd assumed my parents would not have the necessary funds to pay for the uniform and books. My mother and father must have felt powerless to take on the state.

I spent my high school years in yet another Catholic school. Now I was not only stubborn, but stroppy too. My height at twelve was the same as my height now, and I was taller than any other child in my class. It was a good day for me when I'd reduced a teacher to tears. There were two teachers I liked and both of them validated my intelligence and ability to learn. The rest had little or no understanding, and not a lot of interest. They had no way of dealing with my growing resentment and I, in turn, had no respect or anything positive to say about them. I began looking out for any anti-Catholic book I could find and became more and more outspoken.

An interest in boys was developing among my classmates, but I was not a part of the discussions, the jokey conversations, the planning for outings that went on. I'd had friends before high school, but now I was very isolated. I would have liked to have been a part of it all but I never got the chance.

By the time I was fifteen I was a full-blown atheist. I remembered about the black babies we'd been told to buy in earlier years; I remembered about my scholarship and how it had been taken away from me. I told the teachers, the priests, and anyone else who would listen to me that the Pope was not infallible. I'd read about Lucretia Borgia, one of the then Pope's illegitimate children, and she was but one of several. Had they heard about that, I'd ask? I was reading books banned by the Catholic church, and by the time I grasped the full implications of Henry VIII's breakaway from Rome I had drawn the conclusion that all religions were much the same. I hadn't looked at any Muslim religious beliefs, but I had a clear certainty of the hypocrisy evident in Christianity. I saw it all as one big con game.

At home I was talking a lot with my mother. My father's attitude was changing towards me, ever so slightly but changing all the same. His intentions for me were caught up in marriage – the badge of respectability for women, as he and other men saw it. I would then pass from being the responsibility of my parents to being the responsibility of my husband. An antagonism between my parents about religion was becoming more and more evident in the way my mother reacted to some of the school rules. 'You're not wearing long stockings,' she would say; 'you're a young girl, show your legs.' Or 'what do you mean, long-sleeved blouses?' I became a battleground on which my mother fought the Catholic religion and probably, indirectly, my father.

My mother and I spent more and more time together and when I left school at fifteen I stayed at home, helping her. My mother had suggested this and it seemed like a good idea. I think the decision had been made by my parents, but grown-ups had a way of letting you think you'd been part of the decision-making process.

At about this time my family began to visit other families in cities not too far from where we lived and I started to meet other black girls, many of them born into families of black fathers and white mothers. These new friends were thought of as cousins, their parents as aunts and uncles. Participation in social outings and visits was not confined to two adults and their children: when someone's ship came in, it wasn't just his wife and children who'd be there to welcome him but a whole group of people.

The year I was seventeen we moved back to the city. This was the mid-1940s and black American servicemen were arriving on ships with money to burn. With the arrival of those ships the population of black women in the northwest was decimated, as more and more of them went off to live with their new husbands in the USA. Whole families went in some cases. This first exodus was followed by a second when India finally won independence. Then many, many families went to Ghana and different parts of Africa in readiness for independence back there.

I had a wonderful time during those heady years. When people talk about those times now they often convey the message that it was rare for women to be sexual before marriage, but that wasn't the case. It was more that the unlucky ones got pregnant and the lucky ones didn't. I knew that. Other women knew that. I had some sexual experience before marriage and felt good about myself; there was a power about being a black woman. Sometimes I'd make arrangements with three, four, five men and not show up at all. Sex wasn't that good – I have no memory of hours spent in bed with someone who knew exactly what they were doing; it was the buzz around the preliminaries that I remember most. If I think about sexuality during that period, I'd place it in the foreplay of meeting and talking and dancing, not in the bedroom.

I was enjoying my freedom, but slowly, surely that freedom was being eroded. I became more and more involved politically and thought of joining the Communist party, but decided against it when I went on a demonstration in London and learned that racist attitudes were the same in Communism as elsewhere. I should have had a strong sense of my own identity, and in many ways I had, but there was still a feeling that I would have higher status if I married. I fell for it.

The Nigerian man I married the year I was nineteen was not politically involved at all. He was studying, learning about agriculture. I thought of him as a very stable person; I felt he'd pass on some of that stability to me. He was a good bit older than I was and that seemed a good thing too.

We moved to London. This meant leaving the family, so the love and support I was used to was left behind. I felt isolated, cut off: there was no popping in next door or down the street, and visits to other people's houses were by invitation only. It seemed like a different country. I was very lonely and very, very depressed.

Despite my sexual activity before marriage, I was still very inexperienced. Sex soon became a chore. One thing about London was the ready availability of contraception and advice. You didn't have to go to a special clinic or anything like that; every hospital had an out-patients' clinic and information was freely given. It was seven years before I gave birth to my first son.

I'd worked on and off during that time, mostly in snack-bars serving food, though my husband didn't like the idea. I think his love was centred around possession. I made one or two friends through him: previously, up north, I'd had lots of friends, friends of my own choosing, but now it was different. One of these women lost her husband and I spent a lot of time visiting her, talking to her, supporting her. My husband was very resentful and seemed not to understand that this woman needed me. He was acting more and more like an abandoned baby; it was then I realized that though men might grow old I wasn't too sure they ever grew up.

Although there was twelve years' difference between us, I think I was a good twenty years older emotionally than him. I may have been wrapped up in myself and what I was feeling, but he was selfish and became quite doctrinaire. He bought me a sewing machine and then stood over me to watch how well I used it. I became annoyed and told him I was never going to use the bloody machine again. My reading he thought of as evil, and he'd find suspicious motives in the things I said and did. On one occasion at least, though, I had a taste of sweet revenge. I called up the undertakers, told them my husband had died, and asked them to come for the body. I made sure that the time they were due was a time when he would be sure to open the door. If a black man could turn pale, he turned pale that night. I think now that I was always a good mother but a very poor wife. If I'd had my choice, in retrospect, I would have had children and left the husband stuff out of it.

The marriage ended when he left to return to Nigeria. I said I would follow later, but of course I never did. I was afraid of leaving. I'd known a woman who had followed a man to Nigeria and had come back to Britain with only the clothes she wore on her back. We never did get divorced, for six years later he died and that was the end of that. He had married again, I learned later. Legal wives left behind in Britain meant little to him. My son discovered a few years back that he had an older brother in Nigeria, born before my husband came over here. I'd never known about this; there'd not been a word said about previous wives or partners. It was by chance that my son learned of his older brother and it caused him a great deal of worry and concern – mixed feelings of loyalty and excitement.

I moved north after my husband left. It was wonderful to be back in the north. Struggling to bring up my son as a single parent, my confidence was shaky and I felt unsure of the future. How would I cope on my own for the rest of my life? Husband number two soon appeared. He was a charmer, a man from the Caribbean. He had a daughter, much the same age as my son. When finally we got married I knew after just one week that I'd made a mistake. I'd done the same bloody thing twice. I was pregnant with my second son when I knew I'd had enough. I opened the window and threw all his things out; I didn't care where they went as long as they were out of my house. As is often the case, his talk, charming ways, constant chasing after other women were a substitute, a disguise covering his inadequacies. Our love-making had been very disappointing – not even as good as my experience with my first husband. I was glad to be free of men at last and I've been on my own ever since.

I think it's important for children to have a stable environment in which to grow up – I've seen too many unhappy families where men come and go – so I decided to build a strong family unit. My family has been made up of the two boys and me, and a third child I became mother to – my second husband's daughter. Years later, I would ask her if she wanted to track down her mother. I'd help her, support her in the search. No. That wasn't what she wanted. She felt quite content with the way things were.

Separated from my husband, and still pregnant, I sought financial assistance from the state. Even before my first marriage I'd always paid national insurance: I felt then as I do now that independence carries a responsibility and it was important to keep those payments up. The white man who came round to see me was close to retirement. When he entered the house, he immediately commented on the lovely smell drifting in from the kitchen. I'd been making my own bread for some time now and so I explained this and he listened quietly. Something about that bread-making must have impressed him because he told me he was going to do everything he could to help me out. And he did. He set things up in such a way that I got a few extra quid each week, three quid to be exact, for about eight months, until someone back at head office sussed things out and the little extra stopped. It was probably because that man was due for retirement that he'd been willing to take such a risk. That little bit extra meant a great deal to me, and when the bonus did stop I could chuckle and remind myself that I'd had eight months of it anyway. Three pounds was a lot of money in those days.

Those eight months were important in other ways. I'd learned a lot about sticking up for my rights. I'd received maternity benefit when my second son was born, but I'd been carrying him around in my arms because I couldn't afford a pram. Soon I was learning about grants: the pram, laundry and so on. Soon it was the neighbours who were asking me what they were entitled to and I would point out that they could do this or that. It became like a citizens' advice bureau I was running from my home. I became involved in local issues: playgrounds, housing action, black power as it was emerging at that time. Until I retired last year, my whole life was involved with politics, both in my work and in various campaigns such as setting up a black women's centre, women's refuges, education and training, union struggles for pensions and other rights. I would talk to my children about these issues and we'd have long conversations. They attended a small school nearby and I was down at that school whenever I thought it necessary. Like my father before me, I was always on the children's side.

I wanted my children, particularly my daughter, to have respect for their bodies, to use discretion and to think carefully about the choices that lay before them. I'd talked to my daughter all through her childhood and I kept a strict rein on her social life, wanting to know who she was with and where she was going. She had two confidantes and both of these women were very helpful to her, and to me. One of them was my sister, the other a close family friend. I did think it of value that my daughter had somewhere to vent her frustrations, whether or not they were about me.

When my daughter came to me the year she was seventeen and said she wanted to get married, I was at first suspicious. Are you pregnant, I asked? No, she wasn't. She was quite affronted. Her own attitude to sex before marriage proved more conservative than my own. I worry about her future sometimes. Initially, her husband encouraged her to continue studying but it was clear she wasn't interested. She's never worked outside the home and her interests and concerns centre around her family. I'd describe her as working class, though that won't be true of her children. My concern for my daughter is that she might be like the bird in the gilded cage. When the cage is opened, will the bird want to come out? They are a happy family but there's still this question about her sense of identity.

My older son is the perennial student. He's now doing his MA and seems to me to have been studying all his adult life. He does have a child, a daughter, and I was very involved with the baby, visiting the hospital to see the child and my son's girlfriend, doing what I could and looking forward to being a grandmother to a fourth child. But the relationship didn't last and while my son would like to be more involved with his daughter, without the bond of marriage to legalize his involvement, the mother of the child has been quite firm that she wants to break all ties. My younger son, too, is still studying.

If there's a wish that I have for my children and my grandchildren it's that they be given respect and dignity. I would like them to develop and be taught to the best of their potential.

Taking the long way home
Meg Coulson

For twenty years I've lived as a lesbian, reaching this secure sense of my sexuality via a long and tortuous route. Such an identity is not an obvious outcome considering the moral conservatism surrounding my childhood and adolescence, in the 1940s and 1950s Midlands of England. Ironically it was through my most significant heterosexual relationship, begun in my later twenties, that I gained some awareness of other potentialities. Although unexpected contradictions pervaded that relationship it did enable me to move decisively away from the conventions of my family and to make contact with a politics that I could make my own. For my partner, as well as myself, it became a catalyst to further transformations afterwards. But timing, as they say, is everything!

Breaking up, as feminism and gay liberation were breaking out in early 1970s Britain, was timely for each of us. New possibilities were suddenly and astonishingly visible ...

Weddings. I went to so many of them through my twenties. Friends from school and college were marrying, having babies. I was avoiding that. I chickened out of an early possible engagement during my last year at university, extricating myself with an obstinate conviction, but in misery and confusion too. Later I moved away from an 'understanding' with a young man who, like his predecessor, had made himself very acceptable to my family. After that I formed a courteous friendship with a gay man who never acknowledged his sexuality until he committed suicide because of it. The police caught him cottaging and he went home and shot himself.

The atmosphere of sexual morality that I breathed in through the 1950s and early 1960s was narrow, conventional, conformist, promoting self-censorship, suppressing the personal exploration of alternatives. But for all that, for me, it was not totally fixed, unassailable. I grew resistant to those conventions but without a clear sense of where to look for something different.

In childhood and adolescence I was lucky to find several women who fired my imagination in significant ways; women who became for me symbols of something compelling and desirable outside my familiar life. One such idol was a medical social worker – called an almoner in those days – whose thatched cottage in Devon my parents rented for the two-week family holiday for several years. Here I saw an independent woman – she was divorced, had two children – living in a pink-washed cottage with a rambling garden, driving to work each day and coming home to oil lamps and so many books. These summer glimpses inspired my ambition to become a social worker 'when I grew up'. I stuck to this ambition which led me, with very little informed advice, to go on to study sociology at a time when this subject was still fairly unusual. Maybe I sensed more than I could know about this woman who had such an important influence on my life. In her later years she formed a strong attachment to another woman and they lived together into their seventies, devoted companions ...

From my childhood I carried a sense of myself as a sexual being. Despite my grandmother's Victorian strictures when she found me as a small child 'playing with myself', I was not deterred, and masturbated throughout childhood; in fact I have rarely felt cut off from my sexual self. In conversations with my mother when I was about eleven about 'growing up', periods and sex, she was as emphatically positive about sex itself as she was adamant that the only place for it was within marriage. Absorbing both messages I muddled along through my teens and beyond. I took it for granted that I was a sexual being. Yet with boyfriends my relationships were fumbling, sexually and emotionally hesitant and awkward. I was sufficiently enmeshed in the potential for fear or guilt to feel uncertain about what I wanted or what choices I had. I wished that I could feel free of that morality of respectability, but emotionally I was still caught up in it. Knowing that there were other, more liberal ideas was not enough; they seemed too distant, too abstract. Nor were the fantasies I spun around the women I idolized enough; they seemed something quite apart. When, in my early twenties, I felt passionately about a woman I was working with, that also seemed separate. Even now I can recall the dry throat, churning stomach and thumping heart produced by that brief undeclared passion. I must have known, then, that my sexual feelings were involved. Even so, the word 'lesbian', the idea, the reality, existed as a kind of absence in my consciousness. But even as an absence – a space with nothing in it – it was there, enabling me to dodge out of other entanglements.

I had the same kinds of difficulty trying to work out my political identity. Again I had more idea of what I was not than of what I wanted to be. I felt uncomfortably alone, without connection to any living politics that I could identify with. But here again there were clues to work on. By the end of school I was aware of what I was reacting against. All those prescriptions and prohibitions from my family and my white, lower middle-class background, which spilled over into the daily injustices of school life. It was a background steeped in righteous assumptions and strivings for respectability. There was deference to Authority, the Royal Family, God, the Tory party, the sanctity of marriage and its control over sexuality. With my head I despised a lot of that. University gave me access to different ideas – to some theoretical knowledge of Marxism, socialism and sexual diversity but all within a cautious 1950s framework. I found the experience of being a student disappointing as well as intimidating. I ventured to the fringes of CND – ban the bomb – but did not make the personal connections through which I might have come to feel part of that group. Even if I could have made more dramatic links with some of those ideas, I still wasn't ready to make them work for me.

My search for sexual and political identity took a great leap forward in the mid 1960s. I was twenty-seven and teaching social studies in a college of education. I went to a conference in Switzerland, an 'international round table' concerned with youth problems. It was a bizarre experience: a motley collection of 'experts', international conference-goers and young researchers, held in impressive surroundings. There I met Martin.

We spent most of the conference together, walking beside the lake and in the mountains, sitting in lecture theatres and at conference meals. We told of, then replanned our lives. And so I fell in love. I realized immediately, with a clarity and determination that I had not experienced before, that I wanted this relationship. We did not sleep together in Switzerland, each of us in shared rooms and short of money. We allowed such practical obstacles to let us postpone the moment of leaping into bed together. We parted in London to travel home in opposite directions. Already we might have made a commitment to each other, not for life but for as long as love might last. But there was some time for reflection too, the possibility of a different outcome. So we returned to our separate every-day responsibilities. Martin had his uneasy marriage, an apparently fading affair, and his two children to think about. I was freer if I could discount my flatmate, my mother, family and work. And between us stretched 300 miles.

I felt that something quite decisive had happened to me. At last I knew what I wanted. The clutter of conservative constraints fell away. So what if we had to 'live in sin'? So what if my mother would be horrified or even broken-hearted? I would simply tell her that I loved Martin and planned to live with him. I was holding on to the overwhelming sense that this relationship was right.

Then I received a long letter from Martin. It was a kind of confession. I read and reread his words, over and over. He told me he had a neurosis. There followed a careful social scientific account of transvestism (with references to the literature) and a description of his own compulsion to dress in women's clothes. He told me that there was a clinic in Belfast which had developed an effective treatment, an aversion therapy using electric shocks. He was going to make arrangements to go to Belfast to 'get cured'. If I was upset and put off by this revelation he would understand, but he wanted me to know before things went further ...

I *was* shocked. Yet the letter made sense. And I could feel reassured by the honesty of it and even more intrigued by the person who had written it. Rapidly I struggled to understand the meaning of transvestism, drawing on my own social science reading. Suddenly my emerging liberal sexual morality was being put to the test. It felt extraordinary. But all right.

Martin came for a long weekend. I had none of the hesitancy, confusion and ambivalence I'd felt in previous sexual encounters. I was wholeheartedly delighted to be lovers with this person. It was exciting. He was considerate. I even felt that I was quite good at it. He sometimes got very depressed after we'd made love and I found that unnerving, but did not question it.

Travelling became a significant feature of the first year of our relationship and an appropriate symbol of the transition I was making into another phase of my life. Three hundred miles seemed a very long way before the motorways were built, yet weekend after weekend, either Martin or I would be on the road, determined to meet up whenever possible. A nervous energy kept me alert through those lonely journeys; there was the tension of longing to be there and the chance to re-live moments of touch and time together on my way back.

We took the train to Yugoslavia that summer. It was the first (for me) of many visits and the beginning of friendships which have survived the then unimagined personal and political changes. I was stimulated by the differences in culture and politics, the sharpness of criticism and humour, enjoying sunshine and thunderstorms, long and fervent conversations in open-air cafés. Martin and I spent weeks planning an ambitious research project in collaboration with a Yugoslav sociologist; later the research proved to be politically unrealistic and had to be abandoned.

Before the trip, Martin had helped me choose clothes for a hot summer. I was flattered by the intensity of his interest. His own clothes often hung awkwardly, revealing his discomfort with them. It was part of my defiance that I did not care about this or want to change it. I suspect that we both began to adopt a habit of feeling all right if I looked OK. I had never had much confidence about clothes and had focused my attention on looking for unusual shoes. But with Martin's encouragement I grew more daring about what I would wear, more fashionable even. Catching the mood of the times, believing that women should be less self-conscious about our bodies as our skirts got shorter and shorter and shorter, I bought my first bikini. The sense of greater freedom was enticing; I was ready to travel anywhere!

September came and we returned to the realities of living apart. But first there were separate appointments to be kept. I went, without Martin, to my brother's wedding. Dressed up as a bridesmaid, I was acutely uncomfortable, as if these elaborate clothes were a disguise, hiding the person I was becoming. Then Martin set off for the Belfast clinic, with his suitcase full of the women's clothes which the doctors had asked him to bring. He was given a room and a typewriter and asked to provide a detailed account of his life and his compulsion. He awaited treatment. However, since our relationship had begun Martin had had no desire to cross-dress, so there was no active compulsion to treat. At the clinic they told him to come back if and when it returned. I had been playing out horrified images of Martin done up in all the paraphernalia of femininity while electric shocks were administered. It was a relief that this torture was at least postponed. How wonderful if I, and our relationship, could effect such a cure. I felt that this must be a sign of the validity of our relationship. I found reassurance in this secret knowledge.

At Christmas I moved north. I had a new teaching job and I was going to live with Martin. At first we shared the rooms that Martin had been renting in a friend's flat. Later, after a tussle with the building society over my credit-worthiness as a woman, I was able to get a mortgage and we had our own flat at the top of a five-storey tenement block with views across the city to compensate for the climb. All the socialists we knew seemed to live at the top of tenement buildings.

From the start it was a hectic life – work, political discussion, meetings, demos and fundraising, particularly focused around Vietnam solidarity. I had a lot to learn about being politically active in the north, discovering again the sharp differences and inequalities between different parts of Britain, and about the latest debates and analyses, including the fine lines of sectarian disputes. Even social life was political, the late-night parties thick with heavy discussion and heavy drinking. In time we both joined a Trotskyist group, becoming part of the world of the revolutionary left that was beginning to grow in size, influence and optimism. I was inspired by the ideals of revolutionary internationalism, and the interconnectedness of struggles all over the world was made more real by contact with comrades from different countries and continents. While the principles of working-class solidarity and internationalism became wonderfully relevant to me, my grasp of the dynamics of racism (and of class difference too) remained severely limited, even obscured by the revolutionary rhetoric. It was much later that I was challenged into the necessity of developing more awareness of these issues. Gender was not yet on the political agenda of the left either. But despite the imperfections and the gaps in my consciousness, I recognized that I had found a political context.

It was not only the politics. A whole new way of life had opened up to me. Feeling strange in many situations, often out of my depth, I struggled to learn fast, hoping to give the impression of waving not drowning. When faced with the unfamiliar I tended to keep quiet until I could feel that I had collected enough cues to participate. I was far enough away, now, from the influence of family background. And there was scope, despite my lack of a clearly formulated feminist strategy, to work with Martin towards an egalitarian partnership. That he was in a state of reaction to conventional marriage supported this commitment. So we shared shopping, cooking, cleaning, driving, painting; I helped to build shelves in the study in which we each had a desk. I learned to type (slowly) and we wrote and duplicated leaflets, made banners, wrote articles, spoke at meetings.

Our relationship was not perfect. At home I resisted my domestic conditioning, teaching myself not to tidy up after Martin, not to think through all the domestic responsibilities. He was more experienced politically and more effective in political argument (if sometimes too convinced that he had the 'right line'). I did not feel that I ever 'caught up' with him politically, not until our relationship was over. He never did learn from me about plants, birds, gardening or even intuition – that developed afterwards too, and in other ways. But a special delight was escaping together to the country and following the narrowest tracks on the Ordnance Survey map to some remote corner. The monthly visits of Martin's children provided the chance for other explorations of the wild countryside.

I was nagged inwardly by contradictory feelings about Martin's wife. She was having a hard time sorting things out. I held the belief that people ought not to stay together without love, but had little understanding of the difficulties of letting go of relationships, with or without love. I did not feel responsible for the break up of their marriage and the extent to which Martin's wife blamed me for it seemed unfair. Her responses were beyond my influence. I was aware, too, that I never heard her side of the story. There was no outlet for my confused emotions and I became resigned to the moments of isolation and aloneness this brought. Meanwhile I concentrated on developing constructive relationships with the two children and came to care about them very much.

In the bedroom that Martin and I shared, our identities were merging. Only now can it be said that the merged identity was mine. Within that process, I was strongly validated as a woman and as a sexual being. Much later I would realise how far my sense of myself had at the same time been eroded by that experience.

Clothes became more explicitly a feature of our sexual relationship. I did not initiate this development but I accepted it, and enjoyed it too for quite a while. Going to bed often meant dressing up, especially in cheap but silky-textured clothes, and using elaborate make-up. Within our ritual the emphasis gradually shifted. At the beginning I was the one who dressed up, then it was both of us, in soft, silky feminine clothing. Some kind of glorification of the feminine? From the outside of course it may simply look like some gross caricature, but it did not feel like that. It could be arousing, it could be claustrophobic, it could be liberating – all or any of these. And if clothes and presentation are often expressions of sexuality, then perhaps the idea of dressing up for sex and sensuality is less peculiar than it may at first appear?

Through these experiences I began to return to lesbian fantasies, to make them more explicit. My relationship with Martin was nothing like a lesbian relationship but through this ritual celebration of the feminine I became able to acknowledge, fleetingly, the lesbian in myself. I wrote to Sappho's box number and subscribed to Arena Three, a lesbian organization and newsletter run from London in the 1960s and 70s. Discretion and anonymity were still the order of the day; there was no risk of meeting living, self-declared lesbians through taking a newsletter sub; that would require further steps and more courage.

It was the end of the 1960s. We moved to another town, another house, new jobs. A time for changes of many kinds.

Gradually the close sexual identification between Martin and I began to pull apart. Martin now wanted to take on a separate, named female identity, and wanted to venture beyond the bedroom. So he dressed as Martina more and more often when at home.

I accepted Martina's emergence. It seemed to make sense as a further development of the dressing up rituals and the newness of it contained an edge of excitement. But was it my excitement or my absorption of Martina's excitement? I did not know. The strength of our relationship seemed to be proved by its adaptability to significant change and I was reassured by that. Martina became our secret.

But secrecy was a problem. To maintain it we needed heavy curtains, secure locks, and strategies for avoiding unexpected visitors, none of which fitted easily into the kind of political and social life we had established. Against such odds we created an intimate alliance, sharing the secret and sharing the fear of exposure. That made me very tense. But I did not notice what was happening to me. I was getting lost within the isolation of that personal experience, without access to any wider perspective on it, while striving to maintain an appearance of outer calm. In that sense I kept my own cover as much as Martin's.

And I lost earlier insights too, not analysing what was happening when Martin started chasing round (rather ineffectually, I thought) after younger women. In contrast to our combined defence of our domestic privacy, we were quite open with each other about sexual fantasies and adventures. But that was disarming as well, and I remained oblivious to the confusion I was expressing in writing to Sappho and at the same time making more heterosexual moves. I started an affair with another man, a comrade, which became incorporated into the framework of my relationship with Martin. It was sexual but not a love affair. There was room for that but not for the conversation about what it all meant. I became depressed and physically ill.

Then Martin became ill and my strength returned. We were in a state of unacknowledged crisis.

As that autumn ended Martin fell in love. And this was something different. By Christmas our relationship was breaking up. His new lover was a young woman of twenty-seven. I noted the age with wry interest; Martin's wife had been about that age when their relationship began; Martin and I were in our late twenties when we met, and here again he was drawn to a woman of that age. We ceased to be lovers, reorganizing the house so that we could each live independently within it. Our political alliance continued but it was no longer the partnership it had been. Other connections, social and emotional, remained; these would be sorted out uneasily, often painfully, through further changes in each of our lives.

Shocked by the rejection, I wondered what was left of me. At the same time my feelings were so intense, comparable to the intensity of 'being in love'. Everything around me appeared in sharper relief, the colours more vivid, the shapes and sounds more marked — an exquisite misery which lasted for many months. I had to continue teaching, maintaining that appearance of being in control, and I pushed myself into increasing amounts of political activity. The women's liberation movement was stirring and, though conscious of my socialist perspective, I threw myself into its development.

At home we discussed for hours, trying to separate in a comradely way. That was the new moral imperative. (And not a bad one, but how to achieve it?) So Martin and I would talk, Ellena, his new lover, and I would talk. But it seemed as if all the talking had resolved very little. Eight months later I was still struggling. I knew I had to make a decision. I went to London simply to get away. Once there I walked and walked, anonymous amongst familiar landmarks. Trudging for miles along the Embankment, back along the Strand, up to Trafalgar Square and on and on. When I was completely exhausted I caught the train home.

Martin and Ellena were at the kitchen table when I came in. I told her I had to talk to him and Martin followed me upstairs. I insisted that he would have to leave, to move out of the house. The ensuing argument was not rational but full of emotion and anger. I sent Martin's glasses flying across the room. We had never had a fight like that. I was very sharp and clear; he had to move out. And so he did. But still that was not the end ...

That autumn I began a brief period of unambiguous heterosexuality. I saw myself as a political activist, incidentally earning my living by teaching sociology. I drew inspiration from revolutionary women from earlier decades – Kollontai, Krupskaya, Inessa Armand, Rosa Luxemburg – they had struggled on through periods of personal emotional distress; well, so must I! Yet I felt alone, singular, odd ... But I worked hard – late nights, weekends on the move between meetings, conferences, demonstrations – analysing, writing, discussing, organizing. I valued that. Although often critical and self-critical, I believed in what I was doing and that gave me a hold on myself and on my connection to the rest of the world.

My framework for sex was now free love. Over the next months my lovers were comrades. I was not looking for a strong or significant attachment to replace my relationship with Martin. For the time being it was enough to believe that sex could be an extension of working together, with politics very much in command. I did not consider that I was being promiscuous and was startled, offended and hurt when I heard that I had been referred to as a nymphomaniac in some uncomradely quarters. How could I explain my experience and to whom? I was emotionally raw and fragile but I had rescued my sexuality from the dressing up rituals. It was wonderful to do without clothes again, to reclaim the sensuality of nakedness. How far was I aware that I was trying to identify my sexuality once more, in reaction to the latter part of the relationship with Martin? Temporarily I put aside the lesbian fantasies; they seemed too closely associated with that period. I was trying to make sense of what had happened to me. But I hardly talked about it. Much of it was still secret, not out of shame, but who would understand?

Then all around me, secrecy blew out of fashion. The 1970s had arrived. Gay liberation. Lesbians and gay men came out of the closet and for a while the lid lifted on a wider sexual diversity and confusion too. Locally the revolutionary left was reeling as leading comrades made declarations about their sexuality and identity. One gay comrade leaving his marriage rented a room in my house. From that base much gay activity was organized – Gay Liberation Front (GLF) meetings, discos, demos, debates. An exuberant gay scene opened up in the town. Sexual stereotypes, homophobia, bourgeois marriage, monogamy, even falling in love, these were all being sharply challenged. It was an extraordinary time.

In this context of change Martina came out. The identity of Martin was discarded; first by shaving off the beard, wearing make-up, jewellery and uni-sex clothes, then as a transsexual, wanting not only to dress as, but to be, a woman. The public person became Martina – he became she. Earlier gossip and rumour, now disarmingly confirmed, disappeared into the general atmosphere of amazement. Adjustment to and acknowledgement of the new public identity had to be established. The sex-change operation would be arranged at a later date, but the immediate imperative was that everyone should recognize that she had replaced he.

For three months or so I watched GLF's developing momentum from its fringes, drawn towards the atmosphere of excitement and promise that it generated, but hesitant too. Martina had found a safe and validating place. I did not want to follow her there. I had to make my own way and I did so via the women's movement.

During the preceding year there had been an upsurge in feminist activity in the town, including some traditionally styled meetings, actions in support of women workers' struggles, and the beginnings of consciousness-raising groups. Through those months of acute personal distress and uncertainty even the political ground on which I had stood was shifting. And I was changing too. That autumn brought some of the newly visible lesbians to join the women's groups at the university and in the town. It was one of those moments (on a small scale) when politics promises to become a melting pot with unpredictable outcomes. It changed some of the issues for public discussion as well as some personal lives, my own included.

The idea that 'any woman can become a lesbian' may have seemed irrelevant to women clear about their heterosexuality, or even threatening to women holding too fast to conventions of heterosexuality. But it opened doors for me and for many other women. The emerging gay network evolved the means of helping the willing through those doors. The system was simple: spreading information about who fancied whom through social and political circles. It was a rather gentle kind of match-making that minimized the risks of direct rejection and helped the shy along the way. It also allowed you time to know what you were doing. And so after a meal I'd prepared for a few friends one December evening, it was only necessary for the 'significant' young woman to be the last to leave (which she achieved by apparently falling asleep from too much whisky) – and for me to invite her into my bed.

It took me longer to accept myself as a lesbian. I clung to a notion of bisexuality for several months, until I felt that was personally and politically untenable for me. In the end I knew I was a lesbian ... am a lesbian ... have come home. This is my identity. And now I wonder: could I have reached this recognition by any more direct route? The question is, of course, unanswerable. And I remind myself of the ideas, the people, the lives, that I did not know about, that I had no visible means of contact with, when I was younger. Some lesbians know who they are from an early age. I had no such inner knowledge. I had stumbled along, gradually finding clues to a greater political understanding. By a mixture of choice and chance I avoided marriage. Personally and politically I found more coherence through my relationship with Martin, despite my confusion at its end. Eventually I reached the place and the time where being a lesbian became possible to me. And I took that possibility wholeheartedly.

However I did not step into this new life unencumbered. In emotional and other ways many connections with Martina were still unresolved and I did not abandon my sense of special responsibility in relation to her. Rather, I tried to combine these unsettled aspects of the past with a present that was different. This seemed possible in the 'new' moral/political framework espoused within GLF – the rejection of monogamy as proprietorial, the disbelief in romantic love – although, not surprisingly, it created difficulties and resentments that could find no voice. Discrepant feelings were kept in their place, which generally meant out of sight. And I allowed those links to Martina to tug at me.

The children were a significant link. Their monthly visits had continued throughout; we had each continued to see them, co-ordinating the necessary arrangements. At each stage, from the break up between us, to the change of identity, Martina had explained to them carefully and as clearly as possible what was happening, and we both worked to discuss and reassure. The children seemed impressively accepting, and obviously enjoyed their visits and the carnival atmosphere around us.

Then a legal injunction cut all contact. Psychological reports and other professional statements supported the judgment. *No communication of any kind.* Appeals were useless. There was no more contact until the children were legally old enough to make choices for themselves. It was a terrible time. Martina was distraught. I filled up with compassion. There seemed to be no room for my own feelings and responses. These were not my children; I had no claims or rights. Not even the right to be hurt? I pushed my distress away.

I was caught up in other repercussions as well. The press were intrusive, malicious, voyeuristic and, as usual, dishonest. Reporters from one paper pretended an interest in buying a car in order to take photographs after failing in earlier attempts to get interviews or gain access to Martina's house or mine. The Sunday newspaper stories that did appear were nasty pieces in a nasty genre. Presumably they fuelled all sorts of local gossip, but against that I closed my ears. There were other extremely hostile reactions. In one of the worst (for me), Martina and I were forcibly evicted in the middle of the night from a holiday hut belonging to a former friend and comrade. Although rejection and hostility came from diverse quarters I noticed that there was some consistency in the language used: perversion, liability to corrupt, to disrupt the natural order of things, evil influence. These were the recurring themes. And I felt bruised by them too.

Beyond the local gay scene, comrades struggled for a position of liberal acceptance (unsure how to achieve a more revolutionary stance in the absence of any guidance from Marx, Lenin or Trotsky). Old friends divided in their responses. Some reacted strongly against Martina's new identity, feeling a sense of betrayal, not able to perceive or not wanting to find in Martina the person they believed they had known in Martin. Others saw the changes as representing something much more superficial; one Yugoslav friend commented that when they met again she simply had to remember that she should not expect Martina to carry her cases as Martin might have done. There were expressions of admiration as well as revulsion. I picked my way between these differing responses. With a certain sense of mission I tried to stand up for Martina and explain her case to those who did not understand. But this was not always easy to reconcile with my need to verify and consolidate my own position with friends who had previously been 'ours'. For me the unpredictability and inconsistency of other people's reactions became a strain. I was jumpy and sometimes defensive about the rebuffs which seemed to be based in prejudice. I was particularly tense about the lapses (unintended or calculated) when someone referred to Martina as 'he/him' rather than 'she/her', and on occasion when I made this mistake myself I could not own it. I had set myself up as the protector. It must have been from that time that I began to see myself as a rock, firm and supportive through times of change.

I began to monitor the diverse reactions, trying to make sense of instances of tolerance as well as rejection. Martina kept her job and was given a year's sabbatical leave in which it was possible to arrange for the sex change operation and to complete the basic process of transformation. The advantages of an untypically privileged employment, together with the liberalism of the early 1970s must have been important factors here. Through the gay movement I met other transsexuals whose circumstances were more exposed. Working-class individuals, for example, who lost jobs and the usefulness of skills – such as being an electrician or long distance lorry driver – as doctors and employers alike defined these as being inappropriate for a 'lady'. I listened as working-class transsexuals recounted how they had been beaten up, attacked in the street or even at home, especially after some kind of newspaper publicity. These harsh and violent actions seemed to me to express an acute discomfort with any ambiguity about sexed identity, a refusal to consider any overlapping between masculine and feminine, or any complexity involved in movement from one gender to the other (either physically or socially).

Watching Martina's efforts to establish a new public identity, I came to realize that being a woman or a man is not only a matter of physical appearance, of public and personal identity, it is also usually a lifelong experience of being treated in all those so blatant and so subtle gender-specific ways. After all, it is the childhood conditioning, the gender messages received as a girl, the effects of that in adulthood, that I, like so many women, have battled with and against through our lives. These experiences and struggles must be different for transsexuals, for so much of their earlier existence lies outside the now-claimed identity. This extraordinary crossing of the sex/gender divide may provide the potential for exceptional insights into the processes of gender stereotyping and conditioning. But the disparity between past and present may be problematic too, and old legacies may linger on. That general ethical dilemma – can and should any of us deny what we have been? – has a particular edge here. Can transsexuals ever just live in their transformed identities? Must they always acknowledge their past life – or risk discovery of it – with all the uncertainty about acceptance that this may involve? I feel now that taking such a risk must be a condition for the possibility of honesty and trust in subsequent friendships and relationships, and important for personal integration too. That may be the most (politically? ethically?) significant constraint on the process of changing from one sexed identity to the other.

But I also saw the urgency of Martina's insistence, in the early stages especially, on acceptance of her present identity. Initially the women's movement made room for transsexuals like Martina as part of a commitment to sexual liberation, but in the later 1970s this acceptance declined, and in some instances turned into exclusion. I was uncomfortable in the political debates associated with these developments. Seeing too many sides to the argument, I could find no clear political line and knew that my experience had no place here. I rejected Janice Raymond's argument in *The Transsexual Empire* that transsexuals can be seen as part of a patriarchal conspiracy to take over the women's movement, but other issues were more complicated. I could not deny that Martina, like other male-to-female transsexuals, had a masculine past. After all I had lived with Martina as Martin, as a man. That lack of female childhood and past, with the conditioning to go with it, must modify the extent to which male-to-female transsexuals may lay claim to the experience of women's oppression. At the same time, ongoing life as a woman cannot avoid experiences of discrimination or oppression – there's the paradox. It does not seem to be by chance that after Martina's early identification with feminism she later found a more supportive and inspiring framework for her life in New Age ideas and the communities formed around them.

I have become a pragmatist on the subject of transsexualism, taking and accepting the situation as I see it. I do know that Martina has now made both an identity and a life for herself which appear centred and integrated as Martin's did not. Martina can be with herself. Martin never achieved that. At that gut level Martin's transformation into Martina makes sense to me and I value it. I can write that now without feeling that I am on the defensive, standing up for a person and a principle. It has not always been so easy.

Overall my process of unravelling connections to Martina was slow and complex. It must have taken me about three years to begin to question my own sense of responsibility towards her. Eventually I wrote to her to say that I could no longer be relied on for automatic support; we would have to work for a different kind of friendship. For many years, with new friends and old, I would avoid and evade references to this part of my past. I felt that the copyright was not mine; even in my own mind I had allowed it to become Martina's story. It has been good to return, to reflect and to re-examine this period of my life; to share what I have written with a number of friends, including Martina, but to know that I write now for myself.

Through my early years as a lesbian I was simultaneously in reaction to my relationship with Martin/a and trailing strands back to it. In some ways I became more protective of myself. My relationships were non-monogamous and with younger women. This seemed inevitable at the time: simply, I was older than almost all those around me in the local women's community which had grown out of the ferment of lesbian and feminist politics; the critique of monogamy was insistent and convincing. Now wary of investing too much in one other person, I found these ideas attractive. Was I fearful, too, that between women – already sharing the experience of being women – the risk of blurring identities within a sexual relationship might be even greater? At least in non-monogamy none of us expected or was expected to give all of ourselves away.

That, of course, brought other dilemmas and contradictions. The lesbian feminist practice and politics of relationships during that era was full of challenge, earnest and sometimes incredibly optimistic about how we could (or should) change ourselves and the world around us. Such imaginative leaps landed us in new complexities with which few (did any of us?) had the resources to contend. Sisterhood was tautly stretched over the tensions that multiple relationships could generate in the women's community. Within the context of non-monogamy, traditional boundaries between endings and beginnings of relationships, and between friends and lovers, could be positively disregarded. For some women, like myself, multiple relationships really meant that significant relationships overlapped, sometimes for considerable periods, and that some friends also became lovers from time to time. Through this practice it was possible to opt out of some difficulties in a relationship, or to avoid some of the realities of breaking up, although I can only acknowledge that with hindsight.

Fascinating as this might be, this is not the place for an in-depth evaluation of the personal/political issues raised by these lesbian feminist attempts to reconstruct the value systems around sexual relationships. It's enough here to say that, for me, there have been legacies from these experiences which I have slowly recognized in myself and have wanted to address. Fragmentation has been one such issue. There are already so many pressures fragmenting our lives and identities, and for lesbians (and gay men) these are compounded by the never quite resolved challenge of who does/does not know about my sexuality – in how many parts of my life have I come out as a lesbian and who has already 'forgotten' this truth that I have given them? Multiple relationships can bring fragmentation into sexual life – how far is it possible to be open and honest and true to one's whole self in the context of multiple relationships? Struggling with this, my greatest problem was how to go on talking to myself. Non-monogamy, which at first had seemed to offer a way of securing my autonomy, became another way of losing track of aspects of myself. As I have grown older I have wanted more personal integration, and this has meant moving away from the non-monogamy framework.

For more than a decade being older became part of my identity – always older than friends and lovers; always at a different stage in life from those near and dear to me. I drew energy and excitement from these differences but there was also a sense of being stranded. How should I integrate my past with this present? I juggled the gains and the losses, resorting to being responsible, taking it for granted that I should work to try to understand others. Sometimes this was at the expense of explaining or making demands for myself. Where in public politics I saw the necessity of an ongoing dynamic – understanding/challenging/changing things – in my personal life I was stuck for a long time, weighed down by my efforts to understand rather than to challenge or change either myself or the pattern of a particular friendship/relationship. I had turned being older into feeling more responsible. It made me feel oddly solitary. Looking forward in my fantasies I occasionally glimpsed that even odder, older woman that I might become ...

Yet I did not doubt myself in the ways that the younger woman I had been had doubted herself. There were definite principles I was committed to personally, politically, sexually – lesbian, feminist, socialist – and I struggled to make some coherence out of these identities. But how to adapt this knowledge to changing circumstances? I lost ground again. Younger lovers moved on, as I'd known they must, and I was again the monument, the rock that does not change. Why did I not recognize my own ageism in that belief? Why should change be the special preserve of younger women?

As the decade of the 1980s established itself the exuberance of the left faltered, outstripped in radical zeal by the new right. And all of those aspects of identity became problematic in different ways. Was it enough to know myself through a strong sense of personal and political commitments? New questions emerged. Looking forward I saw that feminism might fade as earlier women's movements had done, and that lesbians might disappear from public visibility. Within that I faltered too, unsure how to feel strong as a lesbian without a relationship. That was hard. Living alone and enjoying that, I was also retreating to my 'psychic attic', withdrawing into myself.

I looked for new directions, realizing that I must be different in any future relationship, longing for someone of my own age group. Working hard made me feel exhausted, masking my underlying sense of depression, the weight of being in my later forties. At work I lived in struggles for equal opportunities, against racism, for a worthwhile education, all against the odds. Privately I made myself face the probability that I would not have a relationship again. Indeed I did not expect to find that woman of my own age group, or that she would find me.

As in personal life, so also in the wider political arena, we can make gains and we can be knocked back. When we lose ground in either sphere we never go back exactly to where we were before. The 1980s have not been like the 1950s, although through both decades many reactionary and repressive ideas held sway in Britain. Already the decade of the 1990s promises disturbing times – the demise of the political 'east' in Europe, western military intervention in the Middle East, the rising struggles for democracy becoming entangled with claims for national identity – can this be the emergence of a 'new' world (dis)order? Such unpredictable and turbulent shifts have affirmed my belief that the means of resisting repression, of challenging reaction, have to be re-examined, re-thought. My fear that things would just go backwards (that feminism might disappear, for example) was too simple. The political world is more complex and uncertain than that. If it were not so, the same political formula would work each time. There would be no need for political imagination.

Through my twenties and thirties I was trying to mark out my identity. Mine was a confused search for a political context, for self-awareness and for recognition of my sexuality. Through my forties I was not troubled about how to define myself, but nevertheless sank to great depths of personal and political despair. How to feel strong as a lesbian, feminist, socialist in grim 1980s Britain? I was struck with an overwhelming sense of powerlessness. How to find a way out of that?

Moments of optimism surface in unexpected ways, from the resurgence of struggles against oppression, for liberation and justice, in different parts of the world, from small-scale political victories and local signs of solidarity, from 'chance' meetings ...

When that woman of my age group found me, I recognized her almost at once. With her I have entered a relationship full of positive complexity, in which the struggles for honesty (first with myself and then with her), for commitment and for political engagement have become integral. From her I drew the courage to leave my 'psychic attic' and to close the door on it. I have abandoned the image of myself as a rock, unchanging, overly responsible. Now in my fifties I have rediscovered the will to change, not *who* I am, but *how* I can be myself with greater awareness and greater effect, drawing on these personal and political strands to develop a courage and determination which can contribute, in some small way to the transformation of these unequal times.

Confronting the angel
Patricia Duncker

For Jane Scott-Calder and Shiela Shulman

When I began reading lesbian books no one appeared quite to know what a lesbian was. I read work by women who were undoubtedly lesbian in that they loved women, lived with them and even wrote about the whole experience, either luridly – Radclyffe Hall; coyly – Virginia Woolf; cautiously – Maureen Duffy; or savagely – Jo Jones. I paced across the pages, year after year. Gertrude Stein was easily the most peculiar. Her *Autobiography of Alice B. Toklas* read like a sick joke. Her lover vanished as a lesbian, even as a person; she became the wife of a genius. I had no wish to be either the wife of a genius or even a genius who had a wife. These were not encouraging times.

In 1980 I was teaching *The Merchant of Venice* to a class of undergraduates. I noticed that Antonio was left over at the end of the play. Everyone else had been married off. The year before I had been teaching *Twelfth Night*. Antonio was left over at the end of that play too. He had loved Sebastian with a great passion, risked his life and been arrested, only to see his lover marry a silly, selfish woman. It was obviously the same man in *The Merchant of Venice*, older and no wiser, who was still making the same mistake, loving the young men on the make, risking all and being embarrassedly incorporated into the happily married endings. I saw him quite clearly, at the end of the play.

Antonio at the Feast
The sweet sick air of Belmont stifles me.
Hot nights listening to their chatter,
The irrelevant intrigues, soft kisses, sex.
My shutters stand open on rustling sands –
Lorenzo's girl shrieks, mad with pleasure, somewhere close.

Dogs' eyes follow me hostile in the gardens,
The orchids bloom succulent, torrid with scent.
I spend days watching for ships,
Tideless seas, strangled laughter in the kitchens.

I hazarded my love, lost all I had –
She presides at the feasts, like a witch.
My blonde adventurer, now heavy with jewels,
Their children grinning like gargoyles.

Appropriate, but out of place, I sit perched,
Longing for the swaying ships beneath me.

I am not a poet. I write very few poems. But I use them here because they are my milestones on a long common journey. 'Antonio' was actually an unfulfilled commission for a volume of *Poems for Shakespeare*. Most of the poets who were more efficient and professional, and all of whom were men, did write their poems and had a go at pretending to be Prospero. They had an instinctive sympathy with the powerful. I was interested in the people who were left standing outside when everyone else had gone home.

But I wrote as if I were a man. And a man who loved men. For years I had deliberately separated my sexuality and my writing: who I am and what I write. Men even have the right to love men – over and above a woman's right to love another woman. And to write that love into sonnets, plays, novels. Nobody had any idea what lesbian writing might be. Or indeed feminist aesthetics. The more rashly reactionary would risk statements such as 'There's good writing and there's bad writing...' and somehow feminist and lesbian writing was always bad. It was obviously sensible not to risk writing either. So around the same time I wrote a very brief poem about sexuality in transition.

Tidal Rivers
Ripe with the push of flood tide
The river brims, rank with fertility –
But now on the ebb the mud flats breathe,
Fallow. We both wait for the turn.

And I left it at that.

I had begun to write extended prose fiction. I write prose rather than poetry for the following political reasons. I don't believe that it is possible to write extended verse sequences that are more than collections of lyrics held together by a common theme or meditation. The lyric presupposes the unified subjective voice, even if that voice is able only to splinter and offer fragments. I didn't want the egotism of solitary perceptions. I wanted shared experiences, to know what other people desired and feared. Prose fiction, however modernist in conception, demands an inhabited landscape, inhabited by other people. The lyric excludes other people. The tradition of lyrical writing that we have in English, even when dealing with political themes, argues from single perspectives. The lyric excludes the social process for the sake of one concentrated vision. I didn't want only the moment of intensity, insight and clarity. Even when I wrote lyrics I usually imagined another's perception, another voice other than my own, because I wanted the Other addressed, wrestled with, explained in untidy ways. I was like Jacob, searching for the angel.

The very act of writing is a gesture of arrogance. It is an assertion of self and power. Politically, for a woman, it is decisive. Silence is our great celebrated virtue. We are taught how to listen, condone, deceive. We are not taught to speak the truth.

One of the regional events at the first Feminist International Bookfair which took place in June 1984 was a meeting with Alifa Rifaat, the Egyptian writer. Her new book, *Distant View of a Minaret*, had recently been translated and published in Britain. She spoke little English. I possess no Arabic whatsoever. We talked for about forty minutes. She had astonishing luminous eyes, exactly like those of the ancient Egyptian goddesses, surrounded by hieroglyphics.

'Egyptian women,' she told me, 'weep, weep all the time. This is a picture of my late husband. He forbade me to write. Because he did not want people to say that he was the husband of the famous writer. For fifteen years I could not write.' Her book opens with a stark short piece written from a woman's perspective. Her husband makes love to her in the way that men often do. The experience is nasty, brutish and short. She comes to him with his coffee. He has died of a heart attack. She drinks the coffee herself. 'She was surprised at how calm she was.' It is a fine piece of writing. It has a ring of triumph. And truth.

Alifa Rifaat is a devout Muslim. I have no doubt that she mourns her husband. But I also notice that, in her fiction, as in her life, a man's death has set a woman free. The angel of death is also God's messenger. There was something sinister, liberating and oddly comic about Rifaat's story. The angel of death had come to her as a friend.

Then the angel of death came to me.

A woman I loved died at Christmas, seven years ago. We buried her in the monastery cemetery, within the walls of her enclosed community where she had lived as a nun for over thirty years. The visitors' chapel lies obliquely to the altar and the main body of the church. We never see the nuns after they have entered, apparently gliding on roller skates. They bow to the Host and sweep away down the nave, turning their backs. On that day both the nuns and the visitors wore black and all looked the same; but there were many more of us to mourn her death than there had been of them.

Catholic funerals are lengthy affairs. The requiem liturgy becomes part of the usual Mass. But finally we stood, insecure and distressed, around her golden coffin, singing praises to Paradise. Then we followed the abbess, clutching our tapers, into the cloisters where none of us had ever walked before. As we turned out into the open cloister before the graveyard a damp wind dowsed the taper flames. Then we processed cautiously after the black swaying shapes on to the wet gravel. We were all anxious to do the right thing and be standing unobtrusively in the right place. It is very difficult to behave badly at funerals. Religious ceremonies are coercive and always produce uncannily uniform behaviour. No one howled. No one screamed. No one heard what the priest said into the wind. But we laid her in the earth where she had known she would be buried. 'I'd just prefer a shroud,' she had said to me, 'like the Trappists. They are buried in their habits, and just a shroud. Coffins frighten me. I don't like coffins.' I had agreed then. I do now.

So, for her sisters, she is indeed in Paradise, part of God's continuum which shall continue even unto the last day. And

I, outside the rhythm of their faith, the psalms they sing, day after day, matins, Mass, midday office, vespers, compline, shall never see or hear her again, neither in time nor in eternity. The risk of love is always loss; withdrawal, betrayal, neglect. But the most absolute, irrevocable loss is bereavement. And it is this death and this loss that I have faced ever since, day after day after day.

Death silences even the most brokenly hysterical people. I tell you of my friend's death because I love her still, because I need her, want her back. I have seen people dead, watched my father die, and I have never wanted to shake a corpse and scream, 'speak to me, speak to me', as women do in films. This is because corpses are so utterly unlike the person you have loved. If they have died in exhaustion and pain that death will be dereliction, emptiness, defeat. My friend's death has left me holding my unhealing useless love, unbroken. I have lost my grip on certain kinds of meaning. What does it mean to love when the woman you have loved is dead? You can set up a fund, plan a memorial and continue her work. These are the secular consolations. Or you can pray, pray for her soul in Paradise.

For me, the death of my friend, a woman I loved, has meant a bitter emotional paralysis, but has hacked out the hard space in which to think, and to think feelingly. And so here, confronting my own angels, one of whom is always the angel of death, I ponder the links in my own life between weeping, writing, loving, dying – and how our angels command us to live.

I neither like nor trust men. They are, generally speaking, at best emotional parasites, and at worst, murderous. I do not believe that men are caught in the grip of their biological destiny, and forced by the hormones beetling through their bodies to commit atrocities, consume and produce pornography, abandon or abuse their children and their women. They could choose to do otherwise. But they do not do so. We can all name our honourable exceptions; but men as a group have never organized themselves to dismantle their own self-made privilege over women. They defend as natural, behaviour and practices which have been persistently challenged by women over thousands of years. So that to say that I neither like nor trust men is to say that I can count those I do on a single hand. My friend never contradicted any of this. She simply listened.

Monks and nuns are less likely to recommend marriage and children to the women who come to them seeking silence, spiritual or otherwise. They too stand outside the bourgeois world of marriage and of giving in marriage. They too often encounter the savage roar of disappointment and rage from their families when they refuse to do the decent thing: to buy houses, marry, reproduce the unchanging order. Many celibate religious choose that life because they too are either lesbian or homosexual, cannot or will not challenge the world that would exclude them anyway, and, ironically, find honour, security and legitimacy within a religion that worships the Holy Family. I didn't retreat to the monastery, but to the closet, where I read a lot of books.

My godfather was a Benedictine monk. He was also a pornographer and voyeur, fascinated by lesbian sexuality. He liked to keep in touch with our sundered brethren in the east, the Orthodox Church. He subscribed to *Chrysostom*, their small biannual theological journal. One spring he called my attention to a new book by Elizabeth Moberly, *Homosexuality : A New Christian Ethic* (James Clarke and Co Ltd, 1983). I went so far as to purchase and read this little tract and I mention it here because it has the sublime stupidity supporting the detached ahistorical rhetorical 'we' which is characteristic of most scientific and theological discourse. The analysis the author offers is utterly detached from political realities, completely untouched by feminist thinking, as is the bibliography. To read this kind of text - when I'm feeling sound in mind and limb - feels like watching a gothic folly being built on a motorway. But Moberly's book is not harmless; it is her kind of thinking that dominates a heterosexist and oppressive Church, blights our lives and locks the doors against free women.

Her thesis is simple. Homosexuals - and she makes no distinctions between lesbians and gay men - are sick, sad and immature. Their illness is caused by a 'deficit' in their relationship with the parent of the same sex. This damage is often unavoidable and unintentional. No one is to blame. She carefully avoids any analysis of heterosexual relationships beyond asserting that this is the normality to which we all aspire as mature God-fearing adults. Instead, she redefines the problem. We must separate the homosexual condition from its expression in erotic homosexual acts. We – and here I mean lesbian women – can apparently be cured, by lots of platonic love from another woman and a good soaking in prayer. Erotic encounters are 'a mistaken solution', 'improper', and 'unacceptable'. Homosexuality is the search for parenting; it is therefore essentially non-sexual. With a stealthy flick of the pen Moberly thus casts out of court all possible questioning of the present structure of heterosexuality as an institution; sexual violence against women and children by men, also an institution; and any critical analysis of the difference between female and male sexuality. Lesbianism becomes a state of arrested adolescence. Some of her statements, such as 'Heterosexuality is the goal of human development' must sound odd, even to nuns. But that is by no means the most appalling thing she says. Heterosexuality, according to Moberly, 'is the ability to relate to both sexes, not just to the opposite sex, as a psychologically complete member of one's own sex.' Really? And does each sex relate to the other in the same way? What can it mean to be 'psychologically complete' if, by being so, you have to be heterosexual? And which sex is rendered the object of hatred and desire, the Other, to be exploited, consumed and destroyed? Who holds power in our culture anyway?

Here, Sheila Shulman describes the experience of recognition, danger, liberty, which has also been my experience of lesbianism.

> I felt whole, and could breathe ... I was learning and unlearning at the same time, and I knew I could do both only among women. It seemed to me that I was trying to live in a world that didn't exist yet, that I had to make it, out of nothing and out of buried and silenced bits of the past. I could not make it alone but only with other women who had stepped off the same cliff with nothing but their naked and largely unknown selves. (*Love Your Enemy? The Debate between Heterosexual Feminism and Political Lesbianism*, Onlywomen Press, 1981.)

This is the point at issue. If we question the coercive institution of heterosexuality, with all its trappings of social approval and substantial financial privileges, we challenge the existing order of things. We challenge a Church which regards marriage as a sacrament. If we, as lesbian women, insist on our right to live free, to strengthen and love one another, then we embody that radical challenge. And so we are threatened, abused, persecuted, discriminated against in our work and lives. Many of us give up, give way, give in.

Towards the end of her book, with a great burst of Christian love and charity, Moberly argues that we should be accepted and loved. 'Homophobia ... is unjustified.' Which is preferable to being 'liquidated' – but this is only with a view to being cured and healed of our abnormal tendencies. As most traditional theologians tend to do, she co-opts God on to her side, and appears unnervingly certain of His Purposes. Prayer and love are better than 'medication' because they have fewer side effects. Her finale is a florid swirl of religious rhetoric: 'If we are willing to seek and to mediate the healing and redeeming love of Christ, then healing for the homosexual will become a great and glorious reality.'

Moberly accepts heterosexual practice as 'natural' and 'normal'. Her work floats in a political void; therefore her conclusions that we are pathologically sick and in need of a cure are inevitable. She defines homosexuality as illness. Her arguments are hardly original, but nevertheless dangerous. Her talk of love and healing is hypocritical cant when she cannot see why a world that menaces all women treats lesbians as monsters. Moberly's book was published in 1983. In the summer of 1989 we advertised a lesbian and gay writing workshop in the American lesbian contact magazine, *Lesbian Connection*. We received the following postcard, which I have transcribed verbatim.

> The blood of Jesus Christ cleanses us from all sin. Whosoever is not found written in the book of life will be cast into the lake of fire. The wages of sin is death, but the gift of God is eternal life through Jesus Christ our Lord. Ask the Lord Jesus Christ to save you right now!

Underneath this is written in a different handwriting:

> Homosexual acts: evil perversion by direct choice! 'Vile affections, against nature, lust, unseemly, recompensed error'!

The only people who contradict this kind of thinking are themselves lesbian or gay and intent on finding a space for themselves within one of the central narratives of western culture, that of the Judaic-Christian tradition. I now believe that this search is misguided. There is no place for lesbians in any of the religions invented by men. And I remain sceptical of either inventing our own or rediscovering the Craft. We are uniquely able to unbelieve, to give no credence whatsoever to systems of thinking that demand unconditional assent to irrational feelings. This is a position of strength that we would be unwise to abandon. I never will. But neither will I abandon my friend who has died. Which means that I must try to understand why she thought and felt the way she did. Why we saw different things.

In March 1983 I visited the monastery where my friend lived. A priest I knew was giving a lecture on Cardinal Newman. It was a wonderful performance. His theme was 'Newman and Prayer'. He made both sound humane, plausible and productive; which is no small achievement. Afterwards the nuns asked questions. One woman with a terrifying yellow face said, 'Father, you have given us a very strong sense of Newman's confidence in God's presence. Was there any time in his life when he was acutely aware of the absence of God?' The priest looked at her in some embarrassment. 'Yes,' he said, 'there was. After he became a Roman Catholic and was received into the Church he does seem to have lived through a very difficult time of dereliction and uncertainty.' We all laughed. But I went on thinking about John Henry Newman, a man who had been aware that he did not belong and that he could not shape himself comfortably within the intellectual structures he had created around himself. He was in exile, unwelcome and on alien ground.

Newman in Rome
'The planting of Christ's cross in the heart is sharp and trying...'

It was not as he had hoped.
The old man at journey's end,
Peculiar and embarrassing.

He missed the damp grass in sunlight.
He couldn't speak the language.

Barred heat, fluttered pigeons,
Vegetables brilliant in the gutters.
He haunted the library,
Thought people stared,
Was wretched in the evenings.

The planting of Christ's Cross
In Cardinal Newman
Was a painful affair.
For the first time he saw –
Shaping Darkness, the absence of God.
And the cavernous domes of the Vatican
Enclosing principalities and powers.
Soft rooms hushed with shutters,
Lamps blood-red against the blue.

And now I was watching Cardinal Newman with sympathy and detachment. For I, and many other women, had always lived within the Shaping Darkness. I had never known the presence of God. What he saw for the first time, I had always seen. That summer on the Feast of the Precious Blood I too became a Roman Catholic.

I didn't discuss this decision, made over several years, with anyone at all. My lover would certainly have been appalled. The radical feminist women whom I then called my friends would have considered the deed a form of intellectual suicide; if not sheer escapism, cowardice and betrayal. My mother, brought up among the Plymouth brethren in Devon, still saw foggy clouds of Papist conspiracy floating through history. Her Protestantism, which is the variety I most passionately respect, the savage incorruptible core of clarity, certainty and self-control, shivered with unmistakable distaste. The community of saints is also, and always ever has been, the community of sinners; but for unpardonable, deliberate, criminal wickedness the Catholic Church remains unparalleled. My mother is a historian. I could almost smell the burning heretics.

I do not know God. I find most theology spectacularly irrelevant, both to the question of God and to everything else.

I hated the priests, the rituals, even the Bible, great chunks of which I still know by heart. To me then, it was a more or less unreadable misogynist tract. And so here I must return to my friend who is dead. For without her my action becomes inexplicable, irrational, almost insane.

My friend had never read Marilyn Frye's feminist essays, *The Politics of Reality* (The Crossing Press, 1983), which for me have been so uncannily illuminating. And she wouldn't have needed to do so. The title essay, 'To Be and Be Seen: The Politics of Reality', contains the following passage:

> Lesbians can be seen as not natural in that if someone lives as a lesbian, it is not assumed that that is just who, or how, she *is*. Rather, it is presumed to be some sort of affliction, or is a result of failed attempts to solve some sort of problem or resolve some sort of conflict (and if she could find another way, she would take it, and then would not be a lesbian)...'Being a lesbian' is understood here as certain sorts of people understand 'being a delinquent' or 'being an alcoholic.' ... To see this sense of 'unnatural', one can contrast it with the presumed 'naturalness' of the heterosexuality of women. As most people see it, being heterosexual is just being. It is not *interpreted*.

My friend was a cunning, old, wise woman. She already knew that the heterosexist thinking Frye outlines above is lies. And she wouldn't have been surprised by Frye's concluding definition of who a lesbian is.

> ... lesbians are in a position to see things that cannot be seen from within the system. What lesbians see is what makes them lesbians and their seeing is why they have to be excluded. Lesbians are woman – seers.

And my friend, who was never a lesbian, who was very happily married before she was widowed and entered her order, who had spent all her life healing, learning to discern truth, justice, God, she would have needed no such instruction. She already saw women clearly, and with love. She made us whole.

I will not remember her as she was not. We disagreed violently most of the time, over almost every issue I have raised here. We read different books. She loved spy stories, unspeakably predictable detective thrillers. She thought that John Le Carré was Literature. I queried the category Literature, but begged to differ. We argued endlessly about theology. She believed. I didn't. For all her radical convictions, her beliefs were sinisterly orthodox. But she had only got as far right as the Catholics.

We argued most about the things that mattered most. When she thought I was wrong, she said so. She usually thought I was wrong. But she never stopped seeing me. Or listening to me. Or loving me. Even when we disagreed, I was never misunderstood. And she showed me something I had never seen and had thought was lies: God's unconditional love incarnate, the 'perfect love which casteth out fear.' For the first and only time in my life I saw that the love of women was the love of God. In her passion for the Other, the Angel, the Messenger, my friend had stood waiting for us at the open door. She had refused to slam that door in our faces. She took us in. She listened. She saw who we were.

Men do not see women. They have chosen not to do so. And they have so shaped their concerns and desires that it is now genuinely not in their interests to see us, or to discover who we are. Most women are too busy looking past and through other women in the hope of catching a man's eye to see women whole. They are busy dressing up, painting their faces or performing parts in such a manner that a man will notice them and allow them to be seen – by men. There are sound economic reasons for this and I do not think that these women are fools. But they betray their unseen sisters. And themselves.

Monasteries do not usually bother with mirrors. Someone else will tell you if there's a growth on your cheek, if your veil is not straight or if all your teeth have dropped out. To become an enclosed contemplative nun is, supposedly, to live for and to love nothing but God. This is of course usually very far from the case. Monasteries are worldly places, full of politics, power struggles, incompatible personalities, repressed sexuality and lost tempers. My friend saw this quite clearly. She was not an idealist. But she also saw women – and lesbian women – as the image of God. I do not believe that she is unique, but I know that in her, and in her seeing, I encountered something rare and frightening. That presence was both judgment and love.

My friend died of cancer, in great pain and with courage. In the early autumn the disease was diagnosed. The last time I saw her she was very tired. 'You know,' she said, mocking herself, 'I'm so unspiritual that all I can manage every day are a few psalms.' All that summer I had read Pascal. The *Pensées* were the most irritating theological revelation. He proposed the tactics of contradictory thinking. Try thinking one thing. And if it doesn't work, think the opposite. Think backwards. Look at how the sentence changes if one word changes. Immerse yourself in contradictions and uncertainties. I tried it out. When Pascal died of cancer they found a curious piece of parchment sewn into his clothes. It was the only record of his encounter with God. We have called it 'The Memorial'. Pascal simply headed the fragmented sentences 'The year of grace 1654'.

'The Memorial' is splintered, peculiar, impassioned. It records the time, the date, and the barest surface of his experience, the moment of complete possession. What is clear about 'The Memorial' is its inadequacy. The eloquent manipulator and polemicist of the *Pensées* vanishes; instead he gives us clichés, broken fragments of Biblical quotation, a capitulation to the forms of religious experience, which, when written down, always read like the inarticulate ranting of a maniac carried away by the Hot Gospel. What is also clear is that it was genuine. And that what happened to Pascal on Monday 23 November 1654 changed his whole life. I wrote my own Memorial for Pascal.

The Memorial
See Pascal, choked with cancer,
His body adrift,
Clutching at God.

In the year of Grace, 1654,
Abstract, certain,
Fire, Joy, Peace.

But now he sees only a woman,
Confronting the angel.

I imagined the dying man escaping from abstraction. Instead he sees the woman who is central to Catholicism, the Virgin Mary at the moment of the angel's coming, the image on so many altar-pieces. Then I realized that it was my friend I had seen, my friend facing death. The Annunciation is perhaps the moment in the gospels which has been most effectively appropriated and abused by male thinking. We have seen the Virgin reduced to pretty Christmas kitsch too often to think of her in different terms. And she is the icon handed out to Catholic women: here is Mary, Mother of God, Mother of Sons, the first Christian, pure, maidenly, matronly, full of humility and submission. 'Be it unto me according to Thy Word...' This is the implausible ideal: virgin, wife, mother, the woman who stomachs the consequences and makes no complaint. Go forth and do thou likewise.

I wanted to see the Annunciation as metaphor, as God speaking to woman. For that moment has never been understood, explained or resolved. And I noticed the gasp of fear in Pascal's 'Memorial'. For Pascal never loses control when he is on the ground that he knows, sceptical radical philosophy and theology. But when the knowledge of God came upon him he was reduced to the clichés of Catholicism. His grasp on his own articulacy broke down. 'The Memorial' has been reprinted in Catholic journals as if its meaning is self-evident, and as if Pascal's vision could be shared as common knowledge. This is not the case. His meaning remains obscure, opaque. But, interestingly, one of the Biblical references he cites in 'The Memorial' is from the Book of Ruth: 'Thy God shall be my God.' (Ruth 1:16.) This is a young woman, Ruth, speaking to a much older woman, her mother-in-law, Naomi. It is also one of the few moments in the Bible when one woman makes a passionate declaration of love to another.

My friend died early in the morning of 22 December 1983. She was seventy-four years old. She had been a doctor, a wife, a widow; a nun for over thirty years. She had never borne children. She lived close to her God. But she did not peacefully accept her approaching death. It was her moment of complete defeat. The theological emphasis of Christianity in this century is on resurrection. Medieval theology was obsessed with the God who died in agony. In forgetting that perspective we crucify the truth again. There is no triumph in death. It is the moment, for each of us, when all possibility and meaning end. It is therefore the moment when we encounter God. The moment when we cease to be. The reading at matins on the morning when she died was Isaiah 54.

> Sing O barren that didst not bear; break forth into singing and cry aloud, thou that didst not travail with child: for more are the children of the desolate than the children of the married wife ...

I was one of her children.

What I have written here is the story of a complicated journey, and of the intersection in my life of two warring elements, my Catholicism and my lesbianism. It is also the story of my love for the woman through whom they are linked. Much has changed in my life since she died, but one thing has not and will never change. I remember her. I still love her. I will not give in. I will not forget. And so I am still part of the Catholic Church. Amazingly, I still sit calmly at the back to listen to Mass.

A year ago my neighbour died. He was eighty-seven and had been in terrible pain, waiting for his angel. There was standing room only in the little church for his funeral. The priest got up, the coffin at his feet, and hammered out ten or so fundamental points of doctrine. Then he looked at us all, and said in tones that brooked no dissent, 'And that's the faith.'

We all nodded. Outside it was very hot, and the cut fields stretched away for miles and miles, towards the sea. Each in turn, we walked round the coffin and said our final farewell. The church was so full that I was forced to cling to the altar of Our Lady, my elbow jostling the Holy Sacrament. My other neighbour, aged ninety-seven, leaned over. 'I like your new chickens,' he shouted, being very deaf. That church was full of people who were related to each other, who were jealous of each other's land, who had quarrelled, who were in dispute. We were all uncomfortable and wearing too many clothes. We smelt sweaty and unwashed. We probably all accepted what the priest had offered as the faith on the terms which he had outlined – that is, not as a creed but as a shape: a shape in history, a shape within our lives. I stood there, thinking of my friend. I shall never see her again. I shall never forget her. I shall never leave the Church, because to do so would be to break my promise to her. *Thy God shall be my God.* It is the only link with her that I have left. So it is my task to believe and unbelieve. To remember her truth, even when it is encrusted with lies. And to write down my own.

To live as a lesbian is to live against the stream, to see the world from an oblique angle, to remain bitterly aware that your values are not those of the world which perceives you as a psychological cripple, a pervert, a monster, a threat. Inigo Jones designed the sets for the court masques of King Charles so that there was only one point in the perspective from which the set, stage and audience could be seen entirely, and that place was kept for the king. But only the beggar, cast out from the whole structure of power, can see the king, the court, and the painted stage for what it is. Learning to see as my friend has taught me to see, for her God to be my God, was to see the world again with the beggar's perception: the perception of authority. In the most radical sense she has set me free.

I have no security as a writer, no permanent employment, no independent income. I face the usual risks every woman faces, but I also carry the dangerous understanding of the political consequences of living as a lesbian. My defences are those which chance has given me. I live in rich, western Europe; I am white and educated by the ruling class of England. I have access to information, which is the white woman's frail equivalent of male power. I don't yet crawl miserably across the bottom of the heap. Which means that I can still afford my integrity. And I can still afford to listen to the angels.

Writing, if it is to be in any sense original, is always an exercise in cartography; it is always a journey across unmapped land. The enterprise carries the high risk of failure on its own terms, and the risk of misunderstanding from others. The responsibility I bear is the commitment to intransigence, the refusal to capitulate or to compromise, to give my voice to the unrecognized and the dispossessed. For we are the women on the rim of the circle. We are in the process of becoming. Weep, we have good reason to weep. But write we must, and write whatever the cost. Loving women now, in the last days, is to strengthen ourselves. To enable each other to be. This is what my friend has done for me. And so my theme is grief, grief, loss and rage. I too take the part of the women who weep and curse. I cannot speak for them; but I can articulate our common silence, so that we do not pass by forever, unheard, unwritten, unseen.

Leading a life of my own
Jenny Newman

As a middle-aged woman I choose to regard myself as an intensely sexual being, with the right to express my sexuality in all its complexity. I live with a man I love, and am deeply committed to him; but I don't regard my sexual identity as fixed or static. I see myself at a point of equilibrium, happy enough in the present, on terms with the past and ready to take on the challenging future.

Exactly what that future offers is a mystery. But I have found the confidence to take my chances. Part of that confidence is knowing that sex is for me. I have a song of my own and the right to sing it – loud.

But it wasn't always like this ...

When I was eighteen I entered a Catholic convent in the belief that I had a religious vocation. Five years later I left bitterly disillusioned with my order, the Church and – most of all – myself.

For many years I regarded my early decision to become a nun as misguided, an irrecoverable waste of early life. New acquaintances would remain in ignorance of my convent years unless the man who was then my husband made a point of telling them – when I would grow so embarrassed that the subject was usually dropped as soon as possible. (Even with old friends I avoided discussing it.) And today, at more than twice the age of that unrealistic young woman who decided to dedicate herself to God, I still have colleagues and acquaintances who have no idea I have ever been a nun.

On re-entering the world I was determined to appear as un-nunlike as possible. Dressed with more optimism than taste in a purple Crimplene mini-skirt, black PVC boots, and a wig to hide my scraggy, ill-cut hair, I wanted to present myself as the antithesis of the ex-religious. When in doubt – and I often was – I would deliberately set out to shock.

Underneath, however, the changes weren't taking place as quickly as I'd hoped. Humiliated by my failure, I wanted to put it behind me as soon as possible. But I hadn't learned how to let go of the past. Looking back, I can see that I couldn't hide it from others without disguising some of its most important lessons from myself. As a result of my secrecy I was soon falling into the same old traps.

For example, in the convent my waking hours had been punctuated by a bell shrilling out the time to pray, eat, work, take recreation. Instant obedience to its summons was part of what our novice-mistress called mortification of the flesh – a death not only to sensuous pleasure but to individual tastes and opinions about the way our lives should be organized. I had come to depend on this routine, almost forgetting how to exercise choice.

So, on leaving the convent, I never even paused to savour the possibilities of my new life, but continued to train as a school teacher – the course my superiors had chosen for me – despite my rapid discovery that it was gruelling work for which I had no real aptitude. Within two years I had cut short a period of sexual experimentation by marrying one of my tutors, and predictably began turning to him for a sense of purpose. When ill-health obliged me to resign from teaching, I embarked on a course of postgraduate study in the same department as my husband. Once again, I was demanding the impossible of an institution – for it to make sense of my life for me. Six years' effort and two further degrees did little more than confirm my sense of intellectual inferiority.

My first experience of 'changing my mind' had been so painful that I never wanted to go through it again. It wasn't until everything – marriage, career, hope in the future – had run into the sand that I was forced to consider what had gone wrong.

Breaking the habit of silence has been a crucial part of my journey towards self-discovery. I've pored over old letters and photographs, summoning up memories from the time when I was Sister Lucia. Nothing would make me return to that convent. But without reclaiming those five lost years I could never have begun to live with an understanding of the present and its potential.

Psychiatrists sometimes assume that women claiming to have a calling to the religious life are secretly afraid of sex. I think this view fails to identify the principal attraction of the religious life for many. My own overriding fear was not of men but of marriage. In my small, northern home town there were few women in the early 1960s who modelled alternative ways of life for ambitious young girls. The rows of grey, pebble-dashed houses in the streets surrounding my school represented the only future I could envisage, with me as joint owner-occupier of one such home, a mother with a part-time job if I was lucky.

My early experience of sexual activity was fraught with contradiction. At my Catholic girls' high school we were often reminded that any offence against chastity was a mortal sin. This meant that masturbation, sexual fantasies, or any other gratuitous pleasure in our adolescent bodies placed us in danger of literally burning in hell for all eternity. Once we had 'sinned' the only escape was confession to the parish priest, a prospect more alarming than hellfire.

At the same time, sexual encounters with what was described as the opposite sex were sanctioned – as long as we girls took full responsibility for preserving our own virginity by keeping the situation under control. For me these strictures had two unfortunate results. First, I assumed I could only be sexual as part of a couple; and second, it became my job to control the male sex urge as well as my own. Most of my teenage sexual encounters – outside dance halls, in the back seats of cinemas and cars – culminated in the repeated use of the word *no*, as I plucked groping hands from my bra and waistband. Soon I had grown used to suppressing my own rising excitement. It wasn't until my middle twenties that I relearned how to allow my sexual responses to continue until climax.

Throughout my teens men remained the sole source of my sexual pleasure, and I stayed very susceptible to them. I knew that if I went to university I would soon fall in love. I only wish I'd felt able to ignore all those who preached that sex outside marriage was a sin. As it was, I wanted to be more than a wife and mother, but had no way of discovering what.

I didn't like all the nuns at school, but I did admire their sense of purpose, their belief that no sacrifice was wasted, and above all their avoidance – or so it seemed then – of the boring, routine chores I saw as wasting the lives of other women. Dissatisfied with my chances of worldly fulfilment, and motivated by a mixture of piety, idealism and a desire to excel in that narrow environment, I soon came to believe I had a vocation. Impetuously I announced my decision. The successive waves of apprehension did nothing to shake it. Nor did my piercing regret that I soon would be giving up many favourite activities like sunbathing, reading novels, dancing and riding. Nobody said it was going to be easy. And nobody noticed that I was motivated by apprehension about the future more than the love of God.

Not surprisingly, convent life failed to solve my problems. Soon after I became a postulant I was overwhelmed by a permanent sense of fatigue, despite the rule of an early bedtime. For months I was acutely homesick, and developed an appetite never to be satisfied by the stodgy refectory meals. Not daring to admit to myself that I had lost my way, I interpreted my tiredness, the craving for sweets, and a growing sense of loneliness as requisite sacrifices rather than signs that I was unsuited to the religious life.

It wasn't until after my clothing (the ceremony which marks the novice's acceptance of the habit she will wear from that day onwards) that I was brought face to face with my feelings. Two of the novices in my year were to be sent home. Sister Mary's mother had died, and she was needed in Dublin to bring up her brothers and sisters. Nobody had been told why Sister Kevin had been asked to go. She was an introverted young woman, and I imagine she was judged an unsuitable candidate for an order where openness and simplicity of spirit were far more highly prized than thoughtfulness or independence.

Even though neither woman was allowed to speak about her imminent departure, the distress of these two at being banished from the novitiate was unmistakable. On their last appearance in chapel I studied their tear-stained faces in disbelief. In a few short days they would be free to enjoy everything I was missing. Images of them both getting up at their leisure, shopping for the clothes of their choice, reading a paperback or going to the pictures distracted me from my prayers that night by filling me with envy.

Ironically nobody sent me home, so I plodded on, still convinced my superiors knew best, and that I must have a vocation as no one had told me to the contrary. Despite the monotony and strict discipline of novitiate life other young nuns were patently fulfilled, and I hoped that I, too, would discover the secret of happiness. Meanwhile, I slowly came to see that my attempt to escape the fate of a typical lower middle-class woman had led me into a stronghold of petit bourgeois mores.

As a teenager I had always hated housework, but it wasn't until I became a nun that I found out how domesticity could become a fetish. Often we spent several hours a day cleaning, sweeping, dusting, polishing. In the run-up to liturgical feasts these activities reached fever pitch. Alternatively we worked under the cook's supervision, peeling mountains of vegetables for the adjacent boarding school. How I hated sewing, a lesson avoided in school by choosing Latin instead. In the novitiate to complain would show lack of mortification, so in silence I unpicked my clumsy stitches yet again, as we sat in a circle listening to another novice read aloud from a spiritual book.

Our dedication to manual labour was meant to foster an atmosphere of tranquillity in which we grew daily close to God. So was the emphasis on ladylike behaviour. If we ran, used slang, shouted or slammed doors we had to confess our lack of recollection before our sisters at a weekly chapter of faults (an occasion when nuns acknowledge minor infringements of the rule to the rest of the community). But sometimes the so-called means made the end – Christian charity – difficult to reach. By the end of the second year of my novitiate I was learning how to be genteel while forgetting how to be human.

The convent was on a busy main road. High in the front was a row of small bedrooms, including mine, which had been the servants' quarters in the days when the house belonged to a single family. Late one night we were all woken by a car crash just outside the gates. Clustered by the corridor window we gazed down in alarm. None of the victims was seriously hurt, but several were badly shaken. Clearly we couldn't dash down to help in our dressing-gowns and shorn heads of hair. By the time we had begun to dress neighbours from across the street had gone to the rescue – real Good Samaritans instead of fake ones like us, returning to bed with our privacy inviolate. The modesty that inhibited us from descending without the full protection of our habits was false. I was beginning to feel troubled by these restrictions, but was still reluctant – or maybe scared – to stop and sort things out for myself.

Had it not been for three events, one international and two personal, I might have been there yet, convinced that a life lived according to the Rule was God's will for me, with nothing but a notion of self-sacrifice to see me through.

First came the Vatican Council of 1962–65. It had already ended when I entered the convent, but its ideas took a long time to filter through. For centuries of religious life the emphasis had been on the nun's exclusive relationship with God. During the late 1960s our focus began to shift to the community beyond the walls, and how we might start playing a more active part in it. Nuns started to play guitars, join protest movements, take refresher courses and go on holiday. Our liturgy – matins, vespers and compline – was, like the Mass, no longer to be said in Latin but in English. Most important for me, this breath of fresh air moving through the Church gave many women the courage to leave their convents altogether, an option I had never allowed myself to consider until then.

By the end of my third year my body had grown so inert it felt like a separate entity. I had been taught it was the enemy of the soul, and came to believe it only existed to lug me from bed to chapel to the theological college where I was by now enrolled. Misguidedly I put my reluctance to think about sex down to sublimation rather than lack of energy and repression. My thoughts went something like this: as I'm no longer troubled by longings for men and sex, it must be a sign that I have a real vocation.

But fat and fatigued as it was, my body was wiser than I knew, and from it emerged the first faint signs of an attempt to lever myself out of an intolerable situation.

On the eve of my twenty-first birthday I felt so tired that I asked my novice-mistress for permission to go to bed before supper. All night I lay in a state of exhaustion between sleeping and waking. By morning I was oblivious to the noise of my sporadic moaning at the severe pain constricting my throat. I scarcely heard the rising bell, and spent the rest of the morning in a torpor, struggling to my feet only when told my parents were on the phone to wish me happy birthday, an exceptional occurrence allowed only on that one special day. I then slumped back on to my bed with a raging temperature. Alternate bouts of glandular fever and tonsillitis kept me there for three or four months.

At first I would hear the bell for chapel with an overwhelming relief at not having to answer it. Soon I was sleeping through to eight o'clock, awakened only by the arrival of my breakfast tray, even though I was meant to be following as many observances as possible from my sickbed. I lay inert, my poisoned tonsils leaving me almost incapable of speech, and my energy drained by what I now know was a giant psychological struggle to suppress unacceptable anger at a mistaken choice.

I was far too self-involved to worry about the response of the community at large to my prolonged stay in bed. Sickness was sent by God to try us, so probably they were sympathetic. Personally I counted each moment of illness as a blessed release from a routine that had become intolerable, and had no will to recover. The trial was for those whose job it was to nurse me, running up and down stairs with trays in addition to their usual duties, doing my share of chores, selecting the library books I hadn't had the chance to read for three years but was now allowed during my convalescence, or preparing lighter, more appetizing meals. I did little to spare them. The world had shrunk to fit the size of my sick room, and I had no energy left over to consider those outside it.

My self-absorption was shattered by the second significant event of that time, my father's final illness. I was allowed to return home to see him in hospital for an hour before he died. As a non-Catholic he had initially been mystified by my decision to become a nun. But soon he had grown excessively proud of me, absorbed by what he could glean of convent life. I myself longed not for approval but rescue. However, that felt impossible to ask of a parent with whom I was always at pains to appear happy. I was twenty-one when he died at seventy, and even then I recognized the event as a watershed.

If anyone was going to perform a rescue operation now, it would have to be me. Despite my reluctance to grow up, certain conclusions were becoming inescapable.

By the following autumn I was still feeling tired and weak, but was judged well enough to go to university in preparation for life as a teaching nun. I was sent to a convent in a large northern city, and travelled in from the suburbs to the university every day. At first I felt hopelessly out of place in the English department. I would lumber into the crowded little coffee bar, three stone overweight and swathed in my bulky blue habit, all the more self-conscious for being the only nun in my year. The other students all seemed slim, elegant, vivacious, at ease with fashion and pop music, aiming at jobs I had never thought of for myself – acting, lecturing, journalism. I felt the same sort of envy, or rather yearning, as I had when the two nuns had been sent home from the novitiate. Their lives seemed so full of promise by comparison with mine, and they all looked so poised and worldly-wise I felt far too shy to approach them.

But soon the barriers began to come down. By the end of the first term my twice-daily journey of one-and-a-half hours had proved too much for me. Permission to live from Monday to Thursday each week in a university hall of residence was a milestone. Away from my community for the first time in over three years, I began to tune in to the world at large. My fellow students were reserved with me at first, and I too felt constrained during the first few days in my student flat. But sharing our every-day life we soon began to talk more freely to one another. They would talk about work, politics, clothes and sex, for instance. I would talk about work too – and try to be as discreet as possible about the rest of my life, hidden away in the convent at weekends.

When the recently released film *Women in Love* was recommended to my second-year tutorial group, seeing it became more important to me than anything else. But I was forbidden to go to the cinema without permission from Mother Superior. On this occasion I felt reluctant to approach her. Perhaps this was because she really was the harsh and unimaginative woman I judged her then – or else, with my waning commitment to the religious life, I was becoming increasingly resistant to discipline. Either way, I decided not to risk Mother Bonaventure's refusal, and from this arose the third incident which propelled me back towards the world.

Several student nuns from different orders had been to an earlier showing of the film. The whistles and jeers attracted by their habits had been embarrassing, and they advised me to wear secular clothes. By this time the order had adopted a knee-length habit, so it was easy for me to borrow a matching blue cape of the same length from Natasha, a fellow student, who came with me to the cinema along with her boyfriend, Luke. Just before we parked the car I pulled off my veil. I had enough fashion sense to know that I wasn't everybody's idea of a student, with my thin, lack-lustre hair and thick serge skirt. But at least I wasn't so readily identifiable as a nun. Natasha dashed ahead to join the queue, while Luke and I locked the car.

It was several weeks before I was summoned to Mother Bonaventure's office. Remote and expressionless behind her heavy oak desk, she invited me to sit down opposite her, facing the light. Continuing to scrutinize my features, she asked for an account of my afternoon on Tuesday 23 February. I was puzzled. What was she talking about? Eventually she had to spell it out. Another member of the community had seen me walking between the car-park and the cinema, dressed in secular clothes and holding hands with a young man.

I was very confused. Going to the pictures was wrong, I knew, but why should I be blamed for holding hands with Luke when I had done nothing of the sort? The irony of it all, coming at a time when I felt so utterly asexual. Anger came next, both at the spy and at Mother Bonaventure for interrogating me like this, followed quickly by distress that a nun from my own community should commit an anonymous act of malice against me – either that, or she was suffering from highly distorted vision.

To this day I do not know who reported me to Mother Bonaventure, any more than I've guessed the identity of the convent kleptomaniac who would rifle our few possessions after we had left our bedrooms, stealing any useless items that caught her fancy. At recreation I would scan the faces of the other nuns, half-hoping to detect the misinformant. My efforts were fruitless in all ways but one. As I scrutinized a community which even among other religious orders had a reputation for eccentricity, I came to the conclusion that I did not want to grow old like them.

By the time exams came round I was ill again from exhaustion. Nearly twenty years later I'm still troubled by a recurrent dream dating from that time: I'm back in the convent, and too indecisive to leave it. Life is tolerable but only just. Routine events flicker before my eyes at a speed which tells me that soon I will have left it too late.

In real life I acted swiftly once I knew what to do. Mother Bonaventure readily granted me permission to leave. Nuns who had only taken temporary vows were never coerced into staying against their will, and I had at least another three years to go before my final vows. In my case she seemed almost eager to see the last of me. In general she was an anti-intellectual woman, conservative by nature, and suspicious of anyone whose ideas were likely to change. She gave me enough money to buy two summer dresses, a mac, shoes and tights. Three days later I returned home.

Before leaving I had been troubled — or should I say pleasured — by the intensity of an unprecedented series of erotic dreams where I made love to unknown men. Each time I awoke as my body reached orgasm, an experience then unknown to me in waking life. Clearly a woman's sexual fantasies do not evaporate when she enters a convent. But mine must have been driven deep underground by the rigours of religious life, leaving me too numb to be troubled about sexuality until the time was ripe for me to be able to acknowledge it again.

Soon after my return to the world I was surprising everyone by shrugging off my earlier commitment as fast as I was shedding the excess pounds I'd accumulated over the years. I left in the summer vacation although my vows didn't expire until Christmas. Soon they became meaningless to me, and I proceeded to ignore them long before December came round. Existence on a student grant left me harder up than I had ever been under a vow of poverty, but a heady sense of freedom more than compensated.

I met my future husband on my first appearance in the university in ordinary clothes. We seemed to have a lot in common or rather, he lived the life devoted to books, ideas and music for which I'd been hungering in the convent. When he wanted to end our relationship only two months after I'd been to bed with him, I was too hurt to analyse my own desperate need to cling. Instead I filled the void with a period of reckless and, at times, enjoyable sexual experimentation, and left to travel round the United States as soon as I'd passed my finals. When I landed at Heathrow that autumn he was there waiting for me, saying he'd revised his views about living by himself and wanted to get married. Like me, he was often drawn by what was inaccessible, and inadvertently I'd reawakened his interest by spending the summer abroad.

I admired my husband-to-be for his integrity. If only I'd known that it was too soon for me to entwine my future with any man after so brief a taste of autonomy. Deep down I probably did, but the habit of denying my intuition was too strong to break at this stage. I'd been drawn to my husband in the first place because of his academic expertise and scholarly habits of mind. There was something almost monastic in his dedication to literature. I think he was, in turn, reassured by my convent background. We got on best when I was his postgraduate student, learning my way around his world. After that it slowly became apparent that we were mismatched. I had been schooled to reticence, and my husband proved far too withdrawn to challenge me. He preferred to view me as a dependent. When I began to develop my own enthusiasms and intellectual preoccupations, he retreated for ever-lengthening periods into his study. Even so, we'd been married for ten years before I finally left him. He was very distressed and so was I. The pain brought my feelings on leaving the convent to the surface again, and I couldn't help feeling I'd made the same sort of mistake twice over.

In my teens I had sought a transcendent authority figure – God the Father – who would bestow meaning on every detail of life if I offered myself to him. I now count myself lucky that it didn't work out, but for a long time I was mortified by that failure, trying to disown every impulse that led me into the convent. In the process of 'forgetting' I once again came to depend on an outside authority figure, my husband, for a sense of direction.

Looking back at my early self and learning to accept her, I am becoming all the more determined never again to surrender my autonomy. I am slowly getting better at working out a way of life that doesn't depend solely on other people's expectations, while taking them into account. I still feel angry at having put so much energy into becoming neuter in the service of a religion I now perceive as patriarchal. In the convent I submitted to its male authority figures more completely than I need ever have done in the world outside its walls. As well as a male god and a male pope we had male bishops, priests, confessors and spiritual directors. The founder of my order was a man, and the Holy Rule I was struggling to keep had been his invention. Its trivial prohibitions all testified to the Church's distorted ideal of womanhood: silent, subservient, and too unadventurous to leave the home without permission. The fiat of the Virgin Mary ('fiat' in this context means 'let it be done') was held up as our model response to life all too often: 'Be it done unto me according to thy word.'

As I grow older I suspect that these men placed restrictions on anything likely to ferment female rebellion – strenuous study, 'particular friendships' between women, exuberant laughter, power in the world. Our curiosity was curtailed by what was called in most orders 'custody of the eyes' – visual interest denied by modestly lowered eyelids. Our vow of chastity, I begin to see, was devised not so much for our protection as theirs. When seated in the presence of priests we were not allowed to stretch or cross our legs, and shapeless habits shrouded our figures from their gaze, reinforcing the lesson I had learned first in school: our women's bodies were a source of temptation to others, not of pleasure to ourselves, and if anyone else succumbed to them it was our fault. With our shorn hair, chafing underwear, linen tightly gripping our scalps, long black veils and floor-length habits we were left in no doubt that our flesh was deemed sinful.

From today's standpoint, how can I best turn my early life to advantage? As I ponder my teenage desires and ambitions, I can see that part of what I was seeking in the religious life has relevance for me now. I know that celibacy and autonomy are not necessarily the same thing. But I still have a need for solitude, and try to make room for reflection most days. I dislike materialism, and am gaining confidence to stand out against its pressures in the every-day world, instead of retreating into a cloister more secure in its comforts than most people's homes. Some of my warmest memories of female companionship date from that time, and I'm glad I've had the experience of living collectively with women. I blame the breakdown of trust on the system, not the individuals.

Finally, I am able to acclaim the determination of that misguided teenager that was me to seek a destiny independent of men, money and marriage. When she was ready to take on the world she pushed for change, unconsciously at first. My early life takes its place in a pattern of growth that has defied all attempts – including my own – to stifle it. My present determination to find meaning in experience before doctrine owes as much to my failures as to my successes.

Standing on divided ground
Celia Anwar

I'm twenty-one as I write this, and nearly all my friends have married and settled down; some have even moved beyond marriage to divorce. I alone seem to be rebelling against the idea of an arranged marriage.

Yet I know I cannot easily dismiss my parents' wishes and the issues around my concern to please them get more and more complicated and pressured as time passes.

Although I am very keen to write for this book I wish to keep my identity protected and can only appear in print knowing that my family will never find out.

I come from a family of seven: my mother and father, three brothers, one sister and me. My parents were born in Pakistan. My mother was married the year she turned seventeen and came to England two years later. Both my parents have lived here for twenty-two years, but to see and talk to them you would probably not believe they had been here so long. They are very religious and hold on firmly to traditional and cultural activities, values and beliefs. My father is the stricter of the two.

I attended an all-girls' school for six years. Further education was not encouraged and so most of my friends dived straight into marriage. They were obedient to their parents' wishes and did exactly what was asked of them – got married to a man their parents chose. I didn't believe in arranged marriages at the time I left school and I still don't.

After school, without any encouragement for further education, I gritted my teeth and did an O level course for one year. I gained one pass, in history. My parents' reaction was to discourage me in whatever way they could. I was pushed into thinking that I was stupid, 'thick', and so on. After raging rows that went on day after day, night after night, I went back to college for a further two years to do a pre-nursing course. After successfully completing it I got a job as a care assistant in a day centre, which made me feel independent.

I stayed in that job for eighteen months, and with a weekly wage of £80 my thoughts centred around the possibility of leaving home. I spent every spare minute planning what I'd need to do to make it all possible – making budgets, looking at ads for flats, following up every lead I could. I compiled lists of things I could do without, worked out how much I'd need for rent and bills and what I'd need to get by from week to week, but my wage was simply not enough. Or maybe it was me – maybe I couldn't imagine myself managing on so little? I knew I could scrimp and save on food and other things, but making do without clothes and books would have got me down in the long term. Perhaps my reasoning about finances masked my concern over how I'd manage without the security my family provided. After all, this wasn't just for a week or two and I'd have to face the implications of my parents' response over a long period of time.

Among my friends there's discussion about a wide range of issues, but we all admit that once we are at home it is difficult to speak up or to question things. Too many assumptions are made and too many things are taken as a matter of course. My father was particularly furious when I told him I'd applied to join a one-year Access course for black students at a nearby polytechnic. I decided to ignore his reaction, but I was afraid for a time that he might get so angry that he would hit me. I told myself that if this did happen I'd have to take the matter further. This kind of attitude made it easier for me to hang on to my determination.

Once on the course I made new friends. They encouraged me to talk about my problems at home and were willing to give support and advice. It was during that very important year that I learned for the first time about issues of race, class and gender. I am still learning more about these and related issues.

It was also during that Access year that my mother again raised the question of a visit to Pakistan. The idea had first come up a couple of years earlier and I'd always avoided making any firm commitment, but now it seemed a good idea. The Christmas break fitted in with such a plan and I welcomed the escape from the cold. But I cannot say I was really keen. I kept putting off sending for my passport and in the end it didn't arrive until the day before we were due to leave. My mother had already asked me if I would give up the course if I met a man suitable to be my husband over there. I told her I wanted to finish my course, reasoning that I'd have the excuse of finishing the spring and summer terms before any firm decision could be reached. I was to be away for four weeks. My mother's plan was to stay until the following June.

I changed when I got to Pakistan. I was only there for a short time but I soon got into the role of an Asian lady. I got into the Muslim way of life and the proper Asian traditions. I don't think it was a front; it was real. These were my relatives, and as we don't have many relatives in England it felt very special, a totally different atmosphere. Because I was with relatives who respected me deeply, I had to look respectable for them, which meant wearing Asian clothes and a scarf on my head. If you are totally western over there you are considered an outcast.

I was introduced to a great many cousins and family friends. My mother did not tell me beforehand how many sons there were in each family or anything about them. I met many young men at family gatherings. Some I liked, some I didn't. I learned that men living in Pakistan are remarkably shy; there's a lot of shyness between males and females, especially teenagers. I slipped readily into an easy way of being, and I found it hard to admit that I feel equally comfortable in both countries, that I can adapt to either place.

Not long before I left Pakistan my mother asked if there was anyone I really liked. I told her there wasn't, but when I thought more about it later I decided that there was one boy I had liked. Once back home, my father asked the same question. I began to say no, but then stopped myself. I looked at my father intently. He seemed so desperate to get me married off. He'd noticed my hesitation, so I mentioned the one boy I had liked and we talked about this boy and his family, about what he might do if he came to live over here. In Pakistan he has a business getting spare parts for motorbikes. My father said he thought it might be possible to help get the young man over here; he could be helped to set up a business and I could go on with my course and later get the work I wanted. But, he went on, if it wasn't possible for this young man to come over here, I'd have to be prepared to live in Pakistan. I knew how I felt about that right away. I did not want to live away from England permanently, though I would be prepared to spend some time here and some time over there. Asian husbands are often away working on two- or three-year contracts in places like Saudi Arabia, so they cannot live with their families all the time. The range of work can vary from carpentry to banking and there are so many families involved that it becomes a norm and therefore more easily acceptable.

I was suddenly into the idea of getting married, though only on the basis that if he wouldn't or couldn't come here, I would spend no more than a certain period of time there. It's hard to explain fully why I got so sold on the idea of marriage when I'd been so outspokenly defiant before. I think I felt attracted to the lifestyles I had seen while I was away: husbands seemed to act with great courtesy and respect, and life there looked plush. Plush for over there, mind, not here – there's a big difference and that needs to be understood quite clearly.

My mother was told about the boy I'd liked and she had time to see him over a longer period. She was happy at first, she felt we'd found the right person. Then she learned that he was on drugs and became unsure. We talked about it more when she returned home, and decided to leave it. I was quite sure in my own mind that I did not want to marry a man who had a drugs problem.

But the idea of marriage had been sown in my head and it continues to live on, a healthy plant that I know will grow though I seek to control the spread of it. I know that each year, as I'm getting older, my parents' comments and my own desire to be happy within a marriage combine to make me susceptible to further negotiation about a marriage partner.

My intention is to expand that negotiation as broadly as possible; to include my parents' wishes, as I would truly not want to marry someone they didn't approve of, while arguing for the sort of man who comes nearest to what I feel I want. The further I get towards a career and greater independence the more I realize that I seek a husband who has experience of higher education, the prospect of a good job, a likable personality, and if he's good-looking to boot, so much the better.

I don't expect Mr Perfect but there are qualities that I consider important in both men and women, and if marriage is to be a workable proposition then these things need to be thought about. I was fortunate that things worked out the way they did with the boy I'd liked as I might have married him and lived to regret it. I was more vulnerable to my parents' wishes at that time, and having held out until now I can assume that my strength of purpose will grow. Education has played a major role in developing my confidence and independent thinking on this issue. There are many young Asian women who are not so strong that they can leave home without carrying the burden of family expectations. I feel very aware of the implications for Asian women, whatever choice they make.

I live in the north of England and I'm amazed at what I've seen of young people in the age range of sixteen to twenty-seven in the major cities of the south. I do not feel that they face the same number of problems as those of us in that age group living in the north. Many of the women I know who live in the south come from affluent family-run businesses. Both men and women in those families work and study and have greater access to the world outside the home and the community. As a result, there appears to be more understanding of the motives and wishes of the younger family members. Here in the north far greater numbers of Asian women spend their days at home. Tradition and culture, and the values that accompany them, remain unchallenged. Another difference could be between living in a city and living in a town. The communities I visit in the south are part of big-city living and I note with interest how these southerners take other points of view into account and challenge with openness those things that northern Asians keep contained.

Among my friends there is a lot of mistrust of Asian men. I would not readily choose to go out with an Asian boy. While arranged marriages carry with them some measure of trust from both partners, there is little trust possible in the years of social interaction before a partner is found. I've met Asian men who'll brag that they can marry who they want. They go out with girls for two or three years and then all of a sudden turn around and dump the girl they are with in order to marry a girl chosen by their parents. The girlfriend dumped is most likely a white girl, since going out with Asian girls can present a lot of problems. There would be a great hassle if the girl's parents found out, her brothers might beat the hell out of the boy, and besides, Asian girls wouldn't be able to go to discos or pubs in case someone saw them. The boy might be very upset at losing the white girl he'd been going out with or he may have kept an emotional distance between them, having some idea of the possible future he faced.

I have had a white boyfriend, but it was quite difficult to work out ways to be together. He had Mondays off and I would often skip my polytechnic work on those days when we could manage to meet up. He wanted me to go out with him at night but it proved too difficult even to try. He was Scottish and his attitude around racism was expressed as being akin to the way the Scottish were treated by the English. Once he defended me to some people who went on about me wearing Asian clothes. With him I felt I was simply being myself and that was good, but the struggle around telling lies at home and finding ways that we could spend time together wore me out and my interest faded despite my positive feelings. For example, I knew that if I wanted to see him I'd have to lie to my family. I couldn't ask an Asian friend to cover for me because the chances of my family finding out were much higher, so my excuses invariably involved a white friend, perhaps by telling my parents that I was babysitting or something like that. My parents trusted my white friends unquestioningly. I'm not saying that they wouldn't trust the word of an Asian girl, but there were always means by which they could check out the truth. I had to be so careful and scheming that it got to be quite a strain. It would never have occurred to me to tell my parents about that Scottish boyfriend. I'd have been too afraid of what my father might have done to me.

Though they are proving hard work for me at present, I do care very much about my family. I know I respect their views and would like them to respect mine. But this is where the crunch comes. I want them to understand me within the context of my viewpoint and my choices. I could never imagine myself doing anything that could cause my family shame, but I cannot fit into a mould that is not of my making. It is not the Asian community that worries me but the bond between my family and myself. I need to work out how I can keep that bond strong yet much more flexible.

Things are changing, both here and in Pakistan. One of the ways that racism can be seen as a working assumption is in the view that Asian culture is a fixed culture. Change may be slow, and that applies across culture and traditions, but I do see enormous shifts in the way Asian people view themselves.

I feel that I stand on divided ground when I look at my own life and the future I would reach for. I would describe myself as a westernised Asian woman, and when and if I have children of my own I would not expect that I'd arrange marriages for them, nor would I be upset or overly concerned if they decide to marry a white person.

Stepping out
Sal and Anne

Sal's story
The year I turned seven my world changed. I left home to go to a special school and discovered I was a person with a disability and a new vocabulary to describe myself.

I was born partially sighted due to a hereditary condition known as ocular albinoism, made worse by the fact that my retinas were burnt when I was given pure oxygen a few hours after birth. My uncle made the discovery by passing a lighted match in front of my eyes; there wasn't a flicker. There followed years of visits to specialists, something I stopped at eighteen. No more bloody professionals.

Until I was seven I had just felt different. I was the kid who had hair as white as ice-cream, the kid you gave specific directions to – 'I'm in the kitchen by the fridge' – the kid who had large black letters on her lunch box. I had the easiest seat to find in the classroom, my clothes-peg was at the end of the row, no one would remove furniture or leave things lying around without telling me, and no one would respond to me by nodding their heads. I was the kid who always had the most bruises.

At seven, however, I became a problem because I wasn't learning like the rest of my class. So the professionals stepped in, and in April 1969 I began a new life at the National Institute for the Blind and the Partially Sighted unit at Thomas Street Primary School in Perth, Western Australia, 130 miles from my parents' farm. After Thomas Street I moved on to Sutherland Street. I learned braille and in my last year, aged thirteen, discovered a magnifying glass, something which was not encouraged. Over the next six years I made up for never having been able to read a printed book by cramming in the whole range, from baby books, through children's books and teenage books to adult reading.

At fourteen I moved back home. I was two years behind in school and behaviour, but my body was well into puberty. I had little sexual awareness as far as fantasies or feelings went, but I did know about sex or at least about how babies were conceived, though I didn't quite believe that anybody would be willing to do it. Being at home full time meant I lost the privileges that went with coming home only occasionally. Things didn't go my way so easily and my parents and I began to experience the trauma of adolescence. My former classmates were now two years above me, but I had kept in touch with some of them and basically knew my way around. I was able to hold my own in class and over time was accepted.

The year I turned sixteen I fell in love with Jane, though at the time I could never have used those words to describe my feelings. We were in the same year and spent time together during breaks, after school and at weekends. We frequently stayed at each other's houses and would always sleep in the same bed, though we made the pretence of having slept apart as we knew for some reason we shouldn't. Nothing sexual happened between us.

Meanwhile, I began to put my energies into pretending that Clay was the person of the moment, while Jane really did fall in love – with James, a teacher. I spent this time being awfully cross and not quite knowing why, a situation I resolved in part by deciding to go away to school to do my A level equivalents at the Methodist Ladies College in Perth. After the relative familiarity of a school and classmates I had known since early childhood, the stress of being 'different' began to build up again. I had one good friend at that time – also someone who didn't quite fit because she was Asian. I felt glad no longer to be at a co-ed school and to be away from home but didn't think things through much further. It was a pattern of burying my feelings that continued as I grew older.

In 1982 I started a psychology degree. What became important at this time was personal growth and establishing myself as an independent person. Against the pleas of my mother and sisters, my father agreed to lend me the money to buy a bicycle, which enabled me to go further than college for support. At the same time I began to see myself as having a disability and to question society's part in that. And I started to become aware of myself as a sexual being. Someone had begun to talk about lesbianism, which fitted a vague idea I had about myself but wasn't ready to confront: until now I had pretty much ignored what sexual feelings I'd had.

In May 1983, after having been ill for a couple of months and losing an extraordinary amount of weight, my world fell apart. I felt physically weak and emotionally unable to deal with all the puzzles my mind was coming up with. So I ran. I took six months off, travelling around Australia and thinking as little as possible, ignoring my mind screaming for answers.

The following year I was offered a place on the speech and hearing pathology course I had originally applied for, and felt obliged to accept. Later in the same year I had a bicycle accident, which acted like a catalyst in forcing me to think. For the first time, I thought about who I was and who I wanted to be. I rejected the image forced on me by my parents of a good girl who was going to get a good job. I also decided that at twenty-two it was about time I got rid of my virginity and began to find out about sex by discussing it with anyone who would listen, and by reading. A couple of years previously I had found myself intensely attracted to a bloke called Chris, but unfortunately I had been unable to separate my sexual feelings from an idealised notion of romantic love and he got scared: neither of us was ready to say *it's only lust, so let's get down to it*. This time I wasn't going to make the same mistake, so I found a nice bloke, decided he was *it*, and made sure I stated clearly what I wanted. It was OK, safe, fun, and lasted for three weeks. It gave me yet more confidence: I rejected the idea that being fat was bad and that having a disability was my problem.

On 30 November 1984 I walked into a travel agency and bought a ticket to England. I arrived on 15 January 1985; it was snowing and I knew no one. That year I got my first real job, working for the Youth Hostels Association, and had my first 'real' relationship, which grew out of a good working relationship, a shared history in Australia, and a need in David to rescue someone. It lasted on and off for seven months. That same year I also came out as a lesbian. I was working on the Isle of Wight as an assistant warden and my decision was sparked off by two women who turned up at the hostel one weekend. Something inside me went *wow*, and that was it: I was out and so was David. Being so far away from my family, it was possible not to feel guilty. It also helped that my boss was gay and he gave me a lot of support.

In 1986 I came back to London to work for Feminist Audio Books, a tape library of feminist and lesbian material for blind and partially sighted women. My crude understanding of disability politics became polished and I began a series of jobs in equal opportunities. I had different lovers, lived in different places and learnt to live with my thoughts. I remember admitting to myself and to a close friend that I would probably only have a relationship with a disabled woman if she was partially sighted – a hard one to come to terms with, as I saw myself as pretty right on. Later that year I went to a benefit and was bowled over by a woman. It was lust at first sight and out flew my vow of a period of celibacy. She happened to be a wheelchair user.

As soon as I saw Anne I started to ask friends who she was. Finally someone introduced me. I was in lust, and what registered more than the fact that this woman was sitting in a wheelchair was that she looked young. My resolve of celibacy was ebbing away as I set out to make an impression.

I left the benefit with a kiss and her phone number and it took me two days to pluck up courage to phone her. My reluctance had very little to do with her being a wheelchair user and all to do with my fear of being rejected. We had a brief conversation and agreed to meet the following Saturday, and here we are, two and a bit years later.

I can remember thinking about what we would be up against if we got into a relationship. My thoughts had little to do with how we would make love and a lot to do with where we could go out. Anne couldn't come to my house and what would we do if we were invited to a party and it was inaccessible? I blocked out a lot of my thoughts, and was outraged with friends who voiced the same anxieties.

The beginning was fun. We spent most of our time in bed and friends, family, home and work were neglected. Slowly a pattern began to form in which I was spending most of my time with Anne at her place, very little at home and just enough at work to get paid. What was going on? Why weren't we going anywhere? We spent a lot of time reassuring each other that staying home was OK. It gave us time to talk and we found out that we shared a lot of common experiences about growing up as disabled people. We also spent a lot of time avoiding issues that were beginning to raise their ugly heads. We skirted around my growing anger about never being at home and Anne never being able to come home with me. We avoided discussions about not going out and about being invited to parties that were inaccessible.

One of the things that I have discovered through being with Anne is the importance of being able to go out to the theatre, cinema, exhibitions, together. For me it's about sharing and finding common ground. As our relationship progressed I began to suggest more and more things, but however varied my ideas were they met with little enthusiasm.

I have been given the answers to Anne's reluctance mostly through the experience of going out itself. For example, earlier this year we decided to go to see a film at the Barbican. I rang and got a yes to all my questions about access. The cab we'd booked (which turned up late, so we missed the six o'clock screening we'd planned for and were left with the problem of having to rearrange our return journey) dropped us at the front entrance, where we were faced with a glorious view of the complex from the top of several flights of stairs. How to get down was solved by a man who came up to see what we wanted and then disappeared to get the key to the stair lift. He explained that to get to the cinema we should use the stair lift to level five and then go outside to another lift which would take us to level nine. He added that there were no facilities up there, so if we wanted coffee or a drink we should do that first.

After coffee on level five, a drink on level six and the toilet on level one it was back to level five, only to find that the concourse area had been locked and our way blocked. The response to our question about how to get to level nine was 'take the lift to level eight and walk' – you could have given the man a medal for not noticing that Anne was a wheelchair user. We finally found ourselves following a top security man, who led us up lifts and down corridors, assuring us all the time that the access was fine.

Once on the right level, I left Anne sitting by the door and went to buy tickets. Now it was the usherette's turn to get into a tizz: Anne became invisible and I was told to push her in last; I could sit at the back. Secure in the knowledge that we were going to be able to get into the film, we decided to use the remaining spare time to try to arrange a cab home, which meant back to level three. When I asked the usherette to explain to Anne how to get there as giving me visual directions is useless, she said she would write it down. At this point we began to wonder if we shouldn't just give up and go home.

We stayed. Anne sat in her wheelchair at the back and I was told to sit behind her, to the right. This was no good because I need to be able to ask questions as I find it difficult to recognize faces, which means by the time I've sorted out who's who the film is over. I asked for a chair so I could sit beside her and was refused because of fire regulations, so I got our coats and sat on the floor.

It's not an unusual experience whenever we go anywhere new for me to have a queasy feeling in my stomach about whether the place will really be accessible. If it is, the relief is tremendous. Often I am put into a position in which my disability is forgotten: I am treated as Anne's carer, the one with all my faculties, while Anne is ignored.

Anne and I now live together and experience the same problems as other people who live together. We are managing to do a lot more and Anne, to her credit, allows herself to be hauled up and down flights of steps by me. We have recently succeeded in having a holiday in Hong Kong and the Philippines, and despite the usual hassles (a hotel that had steps up to the entrance and no way of getting to the bathroom) we coped and had a good time. We have learnt that each of us experiences indignity and hurt from such situations but the important thing is not to give up, not to take it out on each other, and to keep trying to live life the way we want to.

Anne's story

I was fifteen months old when arthritis came into my life. My left knee and the little finger on my right hand were the first joints affected. By 1969, when I was two, my left leg had a splint that was removed only when I had a bath, or to exercise. My earliest memories include realizing I had a bad leg and being told I was 'special' because of it. I stopped wearing that splint full time when I was three or four.

On the one hand my family encouraged me to be a 'normal' kid, even down to the beatings I would get if I was naughty; on the other they were overprotective. My mother wouldn't allow me to cross the road on my own until I was fifteen or sixteen, while my brothers, especially the younger one, acted like minders. But my father and I always got on very well. He never hid the fact that I was his favourite, and I never hid the fact that I milked it.

Sex and sexuality weren't serious questions until, at the age of eleven, I was sent to boarding school. The school was for kids with physical disabilities: you know, one of those 'special schools'. The year I started, some of the brighter members of the Board decided it should become a co-ed set up. It was obvious that nobody expected disabled kids to get up to anything of a sexual nature, but they couldn't have been more wrong. They had manufactured a promiscuous society. Within a short space of time I had my first boyfriend.

I was very curious about sex with boys and forgot the sexual fantasies I'd had about women. A vivid memory from my childhood is finding a pile of porn mags in my brother's bedroom when I was about eight. I would go and look at them whenever I could: it was a strange experience because although I was totally enthralled by the pictures, I can remember thinking that women's genitals were ugly, and I was sure I didn't want to grow up looking like that. In retrospect, I recognize I felt sexual, though I didn't understand that at the time and hadn't yet discovered masturbation. I wanted to be a boy and grow up to be a man.

But that all went by the wayside in my first year at school. I had a number of boyfriends and soon began to have sex. I hadn't started my periods so pregnancy was not a problem, which is just as well, because as a Catholic the rhythm method was the only form of contraception I knew. During my first sexual experiences my biggest worry was guilt. I didn't want my mother to find out; I was sure the shock would be too much for her. I was convinced I was in love with everyone I went out with, but I think now that this was an excuse to make it all seem OK.

At the end of my first year I had to go into the hospital I had been attending since I was eight for an assessment. When I went into that hospital I was twelve and walking; when I came out I was thirteen and in a wheelchair. I had been able to walk, run and even ride a bike, but because my posture wasn't good it was decided to operate on my hips. The right hip was done first and it passed without too many problems.

After a boring and painful three months in bed I was given the choice of having my left hip done or starting to walk on my right leg. I chose to start walking, but my physiotherapist encouraged me to change my mind and so I had my left hip done. Even though all the relevant tests were carried out and the doctors knew I had a urine infection, they performed the operation, without antibiotics. Shortly afterwards I started to become very ill, so ill I wished I was dead. I became totally dehydrated and my body was full of poison because my kidneys had failed. Eventually, when I was very nearly dead, it was decided that a drip should be put in my arm and antibiotics given intravenously. I recovered quite quickly, though the delay in starting physiotherapy for my hip meant that it never became strong or mobile enough again. The experience left me with a lot to think about.

As time went on and I was still in hospital I went into a deep depression. I was on a ward for teenage girls and women with arthritis and my only good memories of that time are of the other patients. When I left it was with a feeling that I had discovered true friendship.

I had a week at home and then it was back to school. I fell back into the old routine and started going out with boys again, only this time I didn't waste any emotion, I just got what I wanted out of it. In any relationship the biggest discussion would be where we would go to 'have a bit' – in fact, this was usually the *only* thing we talked about. More often than not we managed – for example, with one particular boy I would go over to the building site that later became the sixth form hostel. The relationships were all heterosexual and I heard of only two cases in which a boy (never any girls) tried it on with another boy.

Of the relationships I had at school, all but one was physical. That one relationship lasted for a year and in the whole time he only gave me two pecks on the cheek. Yet because I was emotionally involved, it was the most important of all. We talked to each other, went for walks, had fun and generally acted like a couple. I was aware that something was missing from my other relationships, but I put it down to the fact that my emotions were all spent, and that I wasn't a very emotional person anyway. In retrospect, I think this was all a big excuse to get away from the fact that it was difficult for me to relate emotionally to the opposite sex.

When we were about fifteen all the haemophiliac boys at the school, of which there was a high percentage, started to use condoms whenever they had sex. I thought how responsible they were being and admired them. It wasn't until I left that I discovered that they had all contracted HIV from the factorate they had to use when they had bleeds. No one else at the school was told; instead, a ban was slapped on sex. Of course it didn't stop us at all, in fact it only encouraged us further. Since leaving school I've heard a lot of these boys have developed Aids and died.

At around this time I decided not to have any more boyfriends because I realized I needed to think and wanted to spend more time on my own. Sexuality was something I had to think about seriously. I was becoming more and more aware of my sexual preference for women and it scared the shit out of me. I had sexual dreams about women that I would try to push out of my mind when I woke up. I was also finding it more and more difficult to control my sexual fantasies about women – something I had had from the age of ten or eleven and had tried to stop. In my last year at school my hatred of 'queers' and 'poofs' took up a lot of my emotional and mental energy, though I now know that all it did was to confirm to people who knew me that I was a lesbian. I kept telling myself that as long as I still fancied boys it must be all right.

I also thought a lot about why we were all at it like rabbits – not just sex but smoking and other things besides. It came to me that I did these things because it was 'normal', that it felt important to keep up with other kids who didn't have disabilities. I became aware of oppression and how the school staff tried to suppress our sexuality. I remembered a time in the hospital when I was told by the sister to stop seeing a boy from the teenage boys' ward. The relationship hadn't been much more than a friendship, but I realize that I had been told to stop because I had a disability.

I began to hate the school even more once I realized what it stood for. There we were, disabled kids in a convenient corner in the middle of nowhere. Why weren't we at home? Our parents had been convinced it was the best place for us. Why? I was too young and inexperienced to work it out, but I knew I was mightily pissed off. I became a very angry and bitter young person. It wasn't until some years later that I realized this was the beginning of my political awakening. I wish I could have used it then in the way I can use it now.

Hospital and school had institutionalized me; at home I felt lonely and alienated, confused and terribly insecure. I decided I was going to need privacy and plenty of time on my own, so at seventeen, before I left school, I put myself on a council housing waiting list. I knew that I needed to establish a base for myself, somewhere where I could have the privacy I craved to discover my identity. I left school when I was nearly eighteen and was able to move into my own place two years later. The freedom and privacy overwhelmed me at first, but it did ultimately have a calming effect, and I became less highly strung than I had been in my teenage years.

Shortly after moving I started coming out to friends as bisexual, which seemed easier than admitting to being a lesbian. I decided I wouldn't just come out, but that I would sound people out first. I was pleased with the general response, which tended to be 'so what?' In fact, despite my attempts to hide it, most people had sussed it already. I was confused because I still felt physically attracted to men. But the point I had been missing was that whereas with men it was physical but not emotional, with women it was both. By twenty-one I was no longer confused. I knew that to be lesbian was natural to me, and was OK.

When I had just turned twenty-two I met, through some work I was doing, an 'out' lesbian. She asked me directly if I was a dyke. I responded by saying I was a bit of both. She was a professional counsellor and I decided to have some counselling sessions. At the time I was still having sex with men but I desperately wanted to come out as a lesbian and knew I couldn't on my own. Through the counselling sessions we became friends and she encouraged me to go out. I had known about pubs and clubs for some time but I hadn't gone to any because I had no one to go with. Having a disability made me self-conscious, and I so desperately wanted to fit in. After all, I had waited so long. The first women-only event I went out to was a benefit for disabled women. I knew it would be accessible and I had the support of friends. It was here I met Sal, my girlfriend. Before I met her I had never had sex with another woman. I had had an emotional but not a physical involvement with someone, but I was nineteen and couldn't handle it, so I just let it fall through. About a year later I had what I can only call 'a bit' with another young woman. It was experimental on both our parts and basically we just kissed and touched each other from the waist up. Sal is still the only woman I've had sex with. We're still together.

My account of our first meeting isn't as romantic as Sal's. I hadn't been 'out' for long and as it was the first time I'd been to a women-only event I was in a state of awe at the number of dykes around me. One thing for sure was that I was a single dyke, and that I was convinced I would stay that way for a long time. After all, no one meets a partner the first time they go to a women-only event, and, of course, I was a wheelchair user and past experience had taught me that disabled people aren't considered to have any form of sexuality. It wasn't until the end of the evening, when Sal asked for my phone number, that I realized she was interested. A couple of days later she contacted me and we arranged to meet the following weekend. Obviously we had to meet somewhere that was accessible and so straight away the pattern of the relationship was set.

Like most new relationships there followed a honeymoon period where physically we learned so much about each other. During this time we had many intimate conversations about each other's childhood and past experiences. It soon became clear that we had a lot in common. I still felt curious about whether, in the beginning, Sal had wondered how, or even if, I could have sex. A little while into the relationship I asked her about this. She answered by saying it had never been an issue for her; in fact the opposite was true, and she couldn't wait to get into bed with me. Needless to say I was pleased by her answer.

The honeymoon started coming to an end two to three months after we met. The major part of that time had been spent in bed. For me it had been great, and relaxing. The strain for Sal, however, had started to show. She was not only physically tired, but mentally and emotionally too. Her work was suffering because she wasn't getting enough sleep. Also, her friends seemed to be getting upset because of the amount of time she spent at my place. I can remember thinking how unfair they were being – wasn't it obvious that she had to come to my place because I couldn't get into hers? It seemed to take a long time for some of Sal's friends to realize why she had to come to my place and not vice versa. These things became issues between us.

We agreed to sit down and discuss how we were going to handle the situation. Sal needed more sleep, which meant less sex. We had a number of arguments over it and grudgingly I agreed that she needed more rest than she had been getting. Once the novelty of the relationship had worn off, I felt embarrassed about my behaviour at that time.

The other issue was the attitude of her friends, some of whom had what I perceived as a stubborn lack of understanding. I was angry and was convinced they resented and disliked me; they made clear the fact that my disability was a problem for them. One of the biggest decisions we made was that if we were invited to a party it had to be accessible, otherwise neither of us would go. I realized then how committed Sal was to our relationship.

We'd been seeing each other for seven months when we decided to live together. Up to that point whenever Sal came round we would stay in. It wasn't that I was content to do so; it was just easier. Not surprisingly Sal started to get restless with this arrangement. Why didn't we go anywhere or do anything? It was my turn to feel pressured. I tried to explain the difficulties I'd had as a wheelchair user whenever I'd gone out in the past. All my experiences had made me apathetic. Also, as a wheelchair user the choice of places to go (especially in the lesbian and gay sector) is minimal. Finding an accessible venue or pub or club is difficult enough, but the problems don't stop there. One of the worst things is toilets. I've lost count of the number of times I've contacted somewhere to find out the access details, been reassured that there is full access, and then found I couldn't use the toilet. It means either I don't drink anything, or (if I happen to be with someone) I sneak outside to the nearest alley or dark corner. It usually ends with a shorter than expected time out and a desperate journey home. And then there's transport. It does tend to spoil a night out when at one in the morning you find yourself waiting for a mini-cab to turn up, knowing that it could be another hour before it does so.

For a long time I was adamant that going out was too much trouble for me but that if it was important for Sal she should go with friends or on her own. Finally she persuaded me. It wasn't an easy or spontaneous process: we always had to plan where we went some time in advance and if things went wrong, always through no fault of our own, we would argue. I felt as if she blamed me because without me she wouldn't have had the problems; I blamed her for making me go out in the first place. It hasn't been like that every time, in fact the bad experiences don't outnumber the good and exciting ones. We have Sal's persistence and optimism to thank for that, and I have to admit that I am more often than not grateful for it. We have reached a stage now where we don't blame each other if a venue is not accessible. It has also made a huge difference that I passed my driving test earlier in the year and now that we've got a car it's our decision when we go out and when we come home. There are times now when it's me who has to badger Sal out of the door.

Sal and I have had many personal problems in our relationship — who doesn't? But what of all the other problems we've had to deal with as well? I mean the problems this society has caused us — the physical barriers of inaccessibility, the patronising and often hostile attitude of some non-disabled people. All this has made it harder for us. We are disabled people having a relationship in a non-disabled world.

It's tough for us but we're strong stuff, we've made it work and we're still making it work. We know that each other and our relationship are worth fighting for.

There's millions of the wee buggers ...
Catherine O'Shaughnessy

It was in the local pub, one Saturday evening shortly after Easter while having a drink with some women friends, that I realized that I was 'late'. I totally dismissed the possibility of pregnancy – or at least, I tried not to think about it – after all, I hadn't any regular sex life, never mind a steady relationship. 'I'm probably anaemic,' I told myself.

During the following week I wasn't feeling too good and this confirmed my notion that I had a bug, which made me take to my bed for the weekend. I returned to work on Monday with renewed vigour, happily awaiting my period next day. It didn't come and I began to have doubts. A home pregnancy test provided both a positive and a negative result. Perhaps my bug was morning sickness?

The questions went round and round in my head. How could I be so stupid as to get pregnant at thirty-two years of age? How could I cope if I was? How would my employers react? How would my family take it? And how could it have happened? There was one possibility which I didn't want to consider seriously.

A few weeks previously I had invited a couple of friends back for a drink after a night out and had ended up with Thomas, a kiss and a cuddle between friends which went a bit too far but stopped long short of penetrative sex. It hadn't even been the right time of the month. From the age of nineteen, when I first experienced sex as part of a relationship, I'd taken many risks, despite the fact that contraception was freely available. If I was going to get pregnant it should have been then, not now at the age of thirty-two. How could I be so unlucky? Then I smiled and remembered something an old friend used to say: 'There's millions of the wee buggers and they can all swim like fuck.'

Seven weeks from the date of my last period, I went to the local doctor, sample in hand. I asked him about anaemia but he didn't reassure me much, instead he asked whether I greeted the possibility of being pregnant with joy or trepidation. 'If I am, I am,' I answered simply. I put the sample in under a false name (that of the Vice-principal of the school I was working in!), explaining that a member of the school staff seemed to have a hot line to the surgery, as the names of pupils who attended for pregnancy tests were frequently bandied about in the staffroom. Having got this far I wasn't so anxious and began to entertain the possibility of being pregnant, despite the problems that would ensue if I was. Occasionally I even found myself thinking that I'd be disappointed if the test turned out to be negative.

I had arranged to phone my doctor three days after my visit to the surgery and on doing so received confirmation of the pregnancy. So that was that. I wasn't over the moon but I wasn't devastated either. I was now sure that I wanted to have this baby and to hell with THEM. I'd get around the problems somehow. I knew there would be pressure from the governing body of the school in which I taught – a Catholic school for girls in a small provincial town in Northern Ireland – to resign: single women teachers were expected to set an example which certainly didn't include sex and motherhood outside marriage. It was an option I couldn't afford if I wanted to keep my baby, and I wondered how many women in similar circumstances had been forced by the various pressures into having abortions they didn't really want. I'd always wanted children and felt confident that my friends would support me. Braced with that positive attitude I set off for Belfast to stay with my close friend Marion for the weekend to talk things through.

Marion was great and said I could share her home if I wanted to have my baby away from the prying eyes of the small town in which I lived. We spent a lovely weekend planning and working out dates. When would I be due to go off on maternity leave? Would I book into a hospital in Belfast or would I have the courage to face 'them' back home? Our main conversation revolved around whether or not I'd tell Thomas about the baby: I felt he had a right to know, but wasn't sure how he'd react – after all, we didn't know each other very well. Certainly from my point of view there wasn't any prospect of a steady relationship even if he wanted one; on the other hand, he wasn't a kid but a mature adult who could share the responsibilities of a child. In any case, if he didn't want to know, then I'd be better off without him.

I returned home that Sunday and rang Thomas to ask him to call round and see me. There's no easy way to tell someone you're eight weeks pregnant, so I just told him straight out. I don't quite know what I expected. I didn't want to analyse all the possibilities; after all, I was trying to be positive.

I suppose he didn't react too badly for a single man nearing forty who lives at home with his mother in a small parochial town and is highly respected by friends and neighbours. He was shocked and kept saying 'you can't be' — it was a bit like playing the Virgin Mary in a nativity play. However, once he got over the initial shock and realized that I neither wanted to get married nor wanted money we were able to discuss things calmly. One thing that hurt was his lack of understanding. I tried to explain how I felt, that he had a right to know and more importantly I had a right to know whether he wished to acknowledge his son or daughter and contribute in any way to their growing up. Instead, Thomas' main concern was that his mother might find out: it would kill her, he said. Calmly I replied that I didn't care if he told his mother or not — I would tell my family eventually. I didn't care about the gossip but just didn't want ever to have Thomas cross the street to avoid me and my pram. We talked and talked and finally he left, still not understanding why I'd told him and suggesting I phone him at work if I wanted to talk to him again, meantime he'd keep in touch to make sure I was all right.

I felt realistic about the conversation: he could have walked away completely; he hadn't denied the responsibility. But he never touched me once. If there hadn't been arms on the sofa he'd have moved even further away, a far cry from the last time he'd been in my home. I knew we weren't madly in love, but we were friends and a friend would have put his arms around me, a friend would have supported me. However, I didn't regret telling him and I knew there was more to worry about than his feelings.

I visited the doctor again and filled in the forms for free prescriptions and collected my vitamin tablets. The doctor said I could leave booking into a hospital for another month to give me time to decide whether I wanted to have my baby in my home town or in Belfast. In the meantime there was a conference I had to go to in England. I was undecided about going, but a woman colleague who knew my secret gave me a pep talk and I decided to go. It was just the sort of support I needed. I met many women that weekend, some a lot worse off than me; they were women who'd gone through difficulties worse than those I was facing. Inspired by what I'd heard and encouraged by what we'd shared, I returned to Ireland refreshed and happy, looking forward to the future.

I could manage, I would get by. I had a good career and a job I liked and I wasn't going to let anybody get me out of that job to satisfy their Catholic morals. Nor would I have an abortion, even though I knew that would be an easier course of action. Oddly enough I became strangely religious in a private way: nothing to do with *their* expressions of Christianity. I reckoned God would help me through the Christian hypocrisy of clergy, convent, Catholic teachers and parents. The kids I knew wouldn't scorn me for very long, if at all. The family members I cared about would also be supportive once they'd recovered from the initial shock.

I'd already found out that I wouldn't have to give notice of maternity leave until after the summer. I reasoned that I would be able to work up until Hallowe'en and, never a slim person, I thought my pregnancy wouldn't be too noticeable until at least mid-September. I had my own modest two-bedroomed house; friends and relatives would help with baby things. Half pay would be a bit of a problem with mortgage, car and loan payments and I'd never been a saver, but probably my family or perhaps Thomas would help. If not, I'd manage somehow.

In buoyant mood I packed the car, heading south to a caravan by the sea to read and knit and watch the power of the wild Atlantic. My sister and her kids were joining me for the July bank holiday weekend and I began to look forward to the time when I could tell my sister about my baby. I knew she would support me but expected her to be shocked, perhaps fearful of the example I was setting her teenage daughters. She'd be concerned about me, about what I'd have to face in my job and in bringing up a child on my own. I saw no point in worrying her too soon; there would be plenty of time.

But that evening I started to bleed. If was just a slight brown stain at first. I didn't worry about it very much, went to bed and slept soundly and it was no worse on the following morning, apart from a slight twinge. I'd been anticipating all sorts of problems, but not this one. Maybe I'd taken too much for granted? What had I done wrong? Was this some sort of retribution?

As the night went on the bleeding got worse and so did the pain. What should I do? The little I knew about miscarriage told me to lie in bed – maybe the bleeding would stop if I did. If I was losing my baby maybe it was because there was something wrong so perhaps this would be for the best? If I lost the baby no one would ever have to know.

By morning I'd convinced myself that I was feeling better and waved my sister and her family off in good spirits. I was glad to be alone, although a little scared. My friend Mary, that same woman colleague who'd persuaded me to go to the conference, had arranged to call that afternoon. She gave me what support she could, but my need to be alone was strong too and when she left I felt both sad and relieved.

I returned to bed and lay there thinking. Then the pain really took over. I've read since that the pain of miscarriage can often be worse than labour and certainly I had never experienced pain like it and hope I never will again. It continued in waves all afternoon, accompanied by heavy bleeding and clotting. I'd gone beyond hoping for my baby, I just prayed that it would end. I also felt very angry. I had been teaching childcare for years and every single text had devoted about one paragraph to miscarriage, as if it was rare. Not only had I been cheated by this lack of basic knowledge but I could see how I in turn had cheated all those girls I'd taught.

The next day the pain had stopped and I felt well enough to drive home. When I rang the doctor I learned there was emergency cover for the bank holiday; after two hours a woman doctor rang back, listened to my description of the symptoms and told me she thought I had lost the baby but there was nothing to be done except stay in bed and put a sample of urine in when the health centre opened again next day. I put the sample in the following morning, a Wednesday, knowing I'd have to wait until Friday for news. My friend Marion was home on holiday and kept me sane, comforting me as much as she could.

When I rang the surgery on Friday afternoon I was told the doctor had gone for the day. Another night of not knowing. Saturday morning, I phoned at ten. The doctor wasn't in yet, could I ring back in an hour? I did, only to hear an apologetic receptionist telling me the doctor had left for the weekend. I just couldn't stand any more and dissolved into tears. The receptionist finally agreed that I could talk to another doctor who listened sympathetically, which calmed me down, and explained that my test showed a positive result, as though I was still pregnant. This, he explained, was probably due to pregnancy hormones still being present in my body, even if I had miscarried. This was a new piece of information. Why hadn't anybody explained this to me in the earlier telephone conversations?

This doctor offered to come and see me and seemed genuinely concerned about me being on my own. Although I knew that he couldn't do anything, the fact that he was willing to come if I needed medical help was everything. I assured him that I'd survive until Monday and would bring in another sample. It was the not knowing that was the overwhelming problem, but now that it seemed likely my baby was dead I felt calmer. Somehow I got through Sunday and arrived, sample in hand, to see my own doctor early Monday morning. After an internal examination he informed me that there was still something there and that he would get me an appointment at the hospital for a scan the next day.

Marion came with me. We sat on plastic chairs surrounded by all the optimistic mums-to-be. I was directed to an automatic dispensing machine and told to drink some orange juice in readiness for the scan. An hour later I was scanned and told that my bladder was empty. I hadn't drunk enough juice. How did I know how much to drink? The doctor, a woman, took my ante-natal card and wrote across it: 'Bladder empty: incomplete abortion? Admit Ward 9', and dismissed me as though it were all my fault. I had started to cry again. Marion produced a nightdress intended for her mother, now a patient in the heart ward of the same hospital. Once I was settled in, Marion caught the bus back to my house to fetch what I'd need for an overnight stay.

Only after my admission was my shattered faith in the NHS restored. The nurses were marvellous, explaining everything they were doing while trying their best to cheer me up. I drank water until I was ready to burst and then was taken for another scan. Again it was methodical and impersonal, but I knew by the muted tones of the conversation around me that the scan had confirmed my baby's death. I was booked in for a dilation and curettage that afternoon. I knew it was essential and just wanted it over as soon as possible.

Apart from being born, ironic that, I'd never been in hospital. I was a little frightened about having the anaesthetic and being led into the theatre and all that, but in no time I was ready and waiting in a corridor. A nurse gowned and masked in green tried to put me at ease by telling me that her husband was from the town where I lived. She asked me what my maiden name had been. I told her that I wasn't married and that's about the last thing I remember except that the anaesthetist's name was Trevor.

Then I was in the lift going back to the ward. I thought they must have called it off and when the nurses and porter told me it was over I burst into tears again and cried and cried and cried. Later I read my chart: 'Very upset on return from theatre.' My baby had died and all they could say was that I was very upset.

The night after I left hospital I met Thomas in the street. I let the friends I was with go on ahead while I talked to him, telling him everything. I insisted he listen to every small detail and this time he did the right thing – he held me and told me that what had happened would always be a bond between us. He assured me he'd call down to see I was OK. He also said he'd been looking forward to having a son or daughter living down the road. Although it was a bit late, I took comfort from the thought that Thomas too had wanted our baby and now felt sad that this baby was dead.

In a couple of days I returned to the caravan by the sea. I felt I had to return to lay the ghost, and face my feelings about it all. But my ordeal wasn't over yet; next morning I awoke with a terrible itch and a greenish discharge, packed the car again, drove back to see the doctor, related the latest symptoms, had yet another internal examination and was given a prescription for antibiotics. The infection, in my opinion, came about because of the length of time I had to wait around before being admitted to hospital. Back to the caravan and sea yet again, but somehow I couldn't settle. I could accept that I had lost my baby but I wanted to know why.

I drove home determined to seek out information. I searched bookshops and libraries for relevant material but discovered precious little on baby death generally, while miscarriage, when mentioned at all, was dismissed as though it were nothing. However, I did learn that miscarriage isn't uncommon; it can be as high as one in four pregnancies, one in two in the first two months. My baby died at twelve/thirteen weeks and I don't know why. Am I ever likely to? Maybe the foetus was imperfectly formed? Was there something wrong with the placenta? Maybe it was something I did unknowingly? The medical profession seemed to think I should get on with my life and try again in three months' time. I was not in a position to try again and wouldn't have wanted to anyway without some knowledge of what had gone wrong.

I went back to work in September and tried to carry on as normally as possible, though I found myself noting pregnant women and imagining what might have been. Apart from Mary, no one at work had known I was pregnant, and in some ways this made it more difficult. In other ways I was grateful not to have to face the problems pregnancy and motherhood would have brought.

I mourned for my baby with a grief like that I experienced after my mother died. Though I eventually gave away the few babies' things I'd bought, in the first few weeks I would often take them off the shelf to look at them and cry. Marion had wanted me to give them to her to pass on, but I knew I needed that mourning period and that those small bits of baby clothes had a part to play. My baby should have been born at the end of January and that time of year will always remain special. As time passes it has become a bit easier. But I haven't stopped thinking about this unborn child and never will entirely.

My initial reaction once the physical and emotional scars had healed was to feel quite proud that I could in fact conceive. Although I didn't set out to get pregnant, I have always wanted children and had sometimes felt that getting married and reproducing was something I was missing out on. Yet was it something I really wanted or just what was expected of me? Perhaps the subtle pressures, the barbed comments about not leaving it too late had got to me. I had begun to wonder what was wrong with *me* – why hadn't any of my previous relationships worked out?

Now that I have been pregnant and miscarried it is no longer so important to have children – it's as if knowing that I am capable of having a baby has taken away that urgent need, the race against time. I no longer blame myself for the failure of previous relationships – if I'd really wanted to get married I would have done, but there was always something missing.

I know too that if I ever decide to have a baby it will be in very different circumstances. If my baby had lived I would gladly have made the necessary changes, but would that child have suffered in the process? During the brief time of my pregnancy I didn't see beyond the difficulties facing me as an unmarried Catholic teacher and the alienation that would bring here in Northern Ireland. But when I see couples and their young children now I realize the tremendous problems I would have been facing on my own. Could I have coped with the isolation? Would I have ended by resenting my child for upsetting my life so completely, curtailing a freedom I've taken for granted for so long? Would I have smothered that child in my efforts to compensate for a father's absence?

As a result of my experience I've learned to value my friends and family more and to appreciate my independence. I have a job I enjoy most of the time, my own home and enough money to live comfortably. I like living on my own. Occasionally I do feel lonely, but it is OK to feel lonely. Casual relationships or marriage wouldn't cure my loneliness if that was the basis for pursuing either.

In the early weeks after my miscarriage I met a kind, generous and sympathetic man who listened to my story of miscarriage and the loss of my baby and didn't judge. He was visiting a friend in Ireland and I had been asked to provide overnight accommodation. Perhaps it was because he was a relative stranger and someone I wasn't going to have to face every day that I found it easy to confide in him. We talked and then I talked more while he listened for long hours into the dawn after our mutual friends had departed.

John wasn't shocked by what I told him and accepted it as part of me. By doing so, he made me realize how insecure Thomas' rejection had made me, and this realization was the beginning of the return of my confidence in myself and trust in others. We began to see each other at holiday times and kept in touch by telephone and letter in the interim. Our relationship developed slowly but surely for three years, at which point we realized that if we wanted it to develop further, one of us would have to move. I did.

Four years on since the experiences described in this story, I am now living in England and working in a state school, where my career prospects are greatly enhanced. The events I have related seem far removed from my present life. Had anyone tried to convince me that the trauma of miscarriage would fade I would not have believed them; now I know it's true. John and I are still together and our relationship continues to grow, though we have no plans to get married or have children. My confidence and trust are fully restored, even strengthened by the thinking I have done I feel I can say truthfully, knowingly, that it's OK to be me.

The things my daughter taught me
Anna Moreton

Early one evening our eldest daughter, Sue, told me she might be pregnant. She was sobbing brokenheartedly. For five days she had been through hell, ever since the party where she had had sexual intercourse for the first time. Later she told me that she had not had anything to drink, knew exactly what she was doing, and had wanted to have sex for quite a long time. She was three months short of her fifteenth birthday. We waited for three weeks to find out she wasn't pregnant.

Her simple statement threw me into a turmoil I would not have believed possible, and caused me to agonize for many months to come. Although I longed to pour my heart out to every friend and stranger I met, I forced myself into a position of silence. This was partly to protect Sue, but it also proved to be a way of punishing myself and suppressing my own feelings. It wasn't until seven months later, with three special friends, that I spoke about it, sobbed about it, and realized how desperately I needed to work through my feelings, turbulent and terrible as some of them seemed.

This is the story of that time, told in the hope that it might help some other mother and daughter to come through such an experience less painfully than Sue and I did.

Physically, Sue had grown up overnight. By the time she was thirteen she looked like a young woman. She wasn't in the least embarrassed by her body, and continued to wander round the house semi-clad. My husband, Alastair, and I both grew acutely aware of this beautiful young girl in bloom, and her sexual awakening, so difficult to put into words, soon had its repercussions on our family life.

Alastair and I are happily married, and had always enjoyed sharing our sexual fantasies. I am bisexual, and have had a close sexual relationship with a woman for several years, something

Alastair knows about. As Sue matured, I found myself having dreams and fantasies involving young women. Sometimes I would imagine myself initiating them into sex, very gently and delicately, and for the first time I found it hard to confide these fantasies to Alastair. When I did – very tentatively at first – he told me he shared my sense of arousal, but found it even harder to cope with. Perhaps it was worse for a man, dreaming of sex with a woman who looked like his own daughter? Did our fantasies amount to incest, we wondered?

After talking it over at great length, we came to the conclusion that our fantasies weren't going to hurt our daughter as long as they stayed at that level. We decided to incorporate our new feelings into our shared sexual fantasies, carefully avoiding any mention of Sue. We also encouraged each other to be honest about any fears that came up. This worked very effectively, and our sex life benefited from the lifting of our anxieties. When I later talked about this aspect of our marriage with close women friends, I saw our decision for what it was: an important step down a difficult and, for us, untrodden path. And all part of having a beautiful, sexual daughter.

I continued to have a good relationship with Sue, and talked to her about sex on a very personal level. My worst fear had always been that she would get pregnant or catch VD, so I had already told her about the available methods of contraception. She had her own copy of *Make It Happy* by Jane Cousins – to my mind the best book written for teenagers about sex – and it seemed to be read repeatedly by Sue and her many friends who came to the house.

Then came the perfect opportunity to talk about the emotional side of things. I was driving us both on a long journey further north to visit her grandparents. Perhaps being able to avoid eye contact made it easier, but somehow I found myself explaining how at her age I'd found it hard to work out a way of coping with sexual arousal – especially as I'd been terrified of becoming pregnant. This was because of the fear instilled in me by my own father: 'If you ever get pregnant,' he used to say over and over, 'I'll throw you out.' So I enjoyed heavy petting, but would always tell new boy and men friends that I drew the line at intercourse. There were only two who kept on trying to make me change my mind, and I soon dropped them. I told Sue about the snags of this form of 'contraception' – if things went too far I used to turn stone cold, and memories of this cut-off point linger on today. I also stressed the fact that although this method had worked for me, she would have to find her own way of coping.

After talking to my daughter that day I'd experienced a tremendous sense of relief. I sensed that she was really listening to what I said, and vaguely remember her re-affirming my hope that she would find her own way. Perhaps my real hope was that she would follow my lead.

So when Sue told me she thought she might be pregnant, it was a bolt from the blue in one way, but not in another. It tore my heart out to hear her say she had thought of running away, or even killing herself. I comforted and supported her by talking as practically as possible, first of all checking with a friend that it was too late for the 'morning after' pill, which it was. Her period was due in three weeks' time and all we could do was wait. I think she went to bed feeling a little easier for having told me.

I didn't calm down so easily. One half of me remained controlled and supportive, while the other was reining in a sense of anger and outrage. Alastair was working away from home that night, so it was easiest to direct this at him, for not being there. I felt as though I'd coped with so many crises on my own through the years and forgot that he had not been away very often and had always been loving and supportive. Swamped by conflicting emotions, I railed at him in my mind through a long and lonely night.

He arrived home the following evening. My plan to say nothing until after he'd eaten went up in smoke the moment he walked through the door. He sensed something was wrong straight away; I met his enquiring look, and out came the dreaded words.

Usually it is me who over-reacts and Alastair who plays things down by being calm, clear and logical, so when he collapsed on me I could scarcely believe it possible; I thought he was having some sort of heart attack. It had obviously come as more of a shock to him than to me. Only a few months before, when I had told him that I felt Sue was ready to embark on a sexual relationship, he had dismissed my fears by contending she was nowhere near ready. His daughter had grown into a woman too fast for him to take in. He was too shocked to face Sue or have anything to eat for the rest of the night.

It was then that my own anger started to erupt – at Alastair for failing to support me and at Sue for doing this to both of us. I found myself storming along to her room and shouting and bawling at her for her utter stupidity and thoughtlessness. Alastair and Sue have always been close, so I really pushed the knife in when I told her about her Dad's stunned reaction, and reported that I had never seen him in such a state in the sixteen years we had lived together. I knew that would hurt her, and I wanted to hurt her a lot.

The anger was pouring out and I felt horror and relief at the same time. I had always thought I was a sexually open person, and here was this demented harridan screaming and yelling at our daughter for causing all this trouble. I also felt bitterly angry towards the boy and his parents. Once again it was the girl who had to pay the price. Sue was stunned, I could see, but maybe also relieved that I had gone into my bawling and shouting mode, with which she had become very familiar over her fourteen years. She calmly refused to tell me the boy's name, remaining adamant that dealing with him was her responsibility.

Over the next couple of weeks my feelings stayed in turmoil. Part of me was proud that Sue was becoming her own person and making her own way, yet I also felt angry at her for daring to do what I myself had wanted to do at her age but hadn't. Of all my emotions, guilt was paramount: guilt that I had let down Sue by behaving, at times, like a punishing, unfeeling person; guilt that I was responsible for her failure to use contraception; guilt that I couldn't have made a very good job of bringing her up, after all. Endless guilt poured in, and because I'd bottled it up it was all the harder to judge how far it was appropriate. Once he'd recovered from the initial shock, Alastair seemed to find it easier. A couple of days later, while we were digging the garden together, he leaned on his spade and said: 'What are we getting so worked up about? We're behaving like a pair of idiots. It's not the end of the world. We must wait and see, and we'll support and love Sue through it all no matter what.'

We spent our half-term holiday – Sue, our younger daughter Louise and me – at my best friend Rosie's, the place Sue had said she'd make for if she ran away. It was the best place we could possibly have been at such a time. Rosie kept the situation in perspective for us both, helping us to see that what Sue had done was perfectly understandable. She was particularly supportive to Sue, who felt able to open up and confide in her.

Sue's period was due towards the end of the week, but despite drinking gallons of the pennyroyal tea recommended to Rosie by a friend as being good for bringing on periods, nothing happened. The following week I was on a four-day residential course; my joy was indescribable when someone walked in one evening with a telephone message for me from Sue saying 'Everything's all right, Mum.' I found it difficult to stop myself from doing a jig on the table. It was three and a half weeks since I'd first heard Sue's news.

This wasn't the end of the story. After a few weeks I talked to Sue about going to a family planning clinic to discuss contraception. Neither of us wanted to attend the local Family Planning Association, so I made an appointment for the young persons' session at the British Pregnancy Advisory Service in Birmingham. Our appointment was midweek, so we had to keep Sue off school with a 'stomach-ache', not telling anyone except Alastair where we were going. Sue was very, very nervous, even terrified, about it all. As we walked up the stairs she was ready to run away, so I reassured her yet again by saying that the counsellor would be sympathetic and supportive. How wrong could I have been?

I had chosen the BPAS because of the excellent help they gave a friend's fourteen-year-old when she needed an abortion. But our own experience could not have been more different. The interview was conducted in a hospital-type room with a bed and instruments in it, and the 'special young persons' counsellor' turned out to be a white-haired woman of sixty. Both of us took an instant dislike to her. Her manner was a mixture of 'Tut tut, you silly girl' and insincere caring.

When she saw us together we discussed the idea of Sue going on the pill (along with my fears of what it would do to her at this age), as well as other forms of contraception. Then she saw Sue alone, and me alone. It ended up with Sue bursting into tears and begging me to take her away from the place. The cold reception, the waiting area where we sat facing a middle-aged couple with no one else under thirty in the room – the whole place was a disaster, and I felt furious.

Sue and I sat in a coffee bar while she calmed down. What stands out in my mind most is her turning to hug me and saying that I was the best Mum in the world, and how understanding and supportive I was in comparison to that woman. It made me realize that Sue had had no idea what the set-up would be, and that I should have explained more.

So we talked about what to do now. The woman had impressed on Sue the danger not only of going on the pill at fourteen, but of intercourse on an immature cervix, and the high risk of cancer in both instances. Sue didn't want to use a cap or anything inserted, so we were back either to abstinence or a condom. When she decided on abstinence for the time being, I heaved a sigh of relief.

About three months went by and life settled down until Sue came into the kitchen one day to announce, in a very aggressive way, that she wanted me to make an appointment with the FPA, as she had decided to go on the pill. I was dumbfounded, but heard myself saying OK. It was her attitude that puzzled me most – so defiant and stubborn. After talking it over, Alastair and I decided to tell her that we didn't want her to have intercourse until she was sixteen. If she was really determined, then it would be up to her to take responsibility for not getting pregnant. We waited with crossed fingers.

Life went on, and my relationship with Sue continued to improve, along with the usual ups and downs. I felt pleased that we'd been able to be clear about what we wanted from her. About a year or so later she met Andy, and started going out with him regularly. Though she was still underage, I casually told her one day that if she wanted to go to the FPA I'd be pleased to accompany her. She thanked me, but said that if she wanted to go, she would either make an appointment on her own, or else she and Andy would go together. Trying to bear in mind how personal our sex lives are, I restrained myself from asking any questions. Sue had grown up in the intervening months, and was much more her own person. I sensed that she was moving away from me, and sometimes felt pleased and relieved, at other times saddened. Occasionally I would wake up in the middle of the night and worry, but deep down I sensed that it would be all right.

When Aids hit the headlines, I decided to talk with Sue about it, explaining that I wasn't prying, but that if by any chance she and Andy were having intercourse and she was on the pill, would she consider also using a condom? I said I didn't particularly want to know one way or the other, but just wanted her to realize the implications of HIV transmission for herself. To my great joy she told me she had been on the pill for months and had wanted to tell me earlier, but didn't dare. She and Andy had talked about Aids and what they should do, and had come to the same conclusion. I will never forget us sitting on the bed together, cuddling one another and crying, each saying how much we loved one another, and seeing what a long way we had come. I walked out of her room feeling ten feet tall and so very proud of our daughter.

A year later, after putting on a lot of weight and having terrible headaches, Sue discussed coming off the pill. We practised what she would say to the doctor – not *asking* if she should come off the pill, but *telling* him that this was what she wanted to do and explaining she and Andy were using condoms instead. My pride and admiration for her grew. Such courage, such strength and determination.

When one of the editors of this book suggested that Sue and I both write our stories, I was filled with inspiration and fear: inspired to share our experience with others; fearful of looking too closely at what happened and the feelings we might uncover. It took me many weeks to pluck up courage even to mention it to Sue.

In the end, Sue decided not to write her story: the experience, she said, had been too distressing and it was time to put it behind her. I know her article would have been very different from mine, but the fact that we have talked several times about what happened, our feelings then and now, is still a bonus.

As our younger daughter, Louise, comes up to the same time in her life, I tell myself that it will be different for her. We have talked about contraception, and I have been told in no uncertain terms that she knows all she wants to know, and if she doesn't is quite capable of finding out and deciding for herself. She is a much more private and independent person than Sue was at the same age.

Over this summer Sue and I have had several trips out together, and my heart has overflowed again and again when she has linked arms and hugged me to her and said, 'I love you, Mum – you're my best friend.' She has never told me the name of the boy who she thought once had made her pregnant, not even in those dark and angry moments when I ranted at her that it was totally unfair that we should have to cope with all the trauma while he and his family got off scot free. She was right and I was wrong. It would only have caused trouble.

Sue has taught me a lot about myself, as well as what it's like to be young in today's world. It still causes me great pain when I think of what I said to her when the 'Victorian Me' took over and it wasn't until much later that I was able to apologize, and to explain that my reaction had been mixed up with my own fears as a teenager, that it is what my parents would have done, and there was I doing the same to her. Our experiences have given me a new sense of perspective, and I am beginning to realize there are no right answers, particularly to the sticky questions of sex and sexuality. It's also good to see the trust that has grown between Sue and Alastair – we've all learnt so much, and nothing can take that away.

Bi-o-logical
Maggie Sansam

I'm a thirty-seven-year-old bisexual woman. The first person I had sex with was a man, when I was eighteen, and the next person was a woman when I was nineteen. It could just as easily have been the other way round. Since then I've had sex with rather more men than women, which is probably due to a combination of things. I hate 'the scene', so I tend not to meet the same number of receptive women as I do men. Also, of course, you're always perceived as straight unless you make a point of emphasizing otherwise – so predictably I get more overt interest from men than from women.

I think I've always felt that sexuality is far from fixed. I believe that if society didn't place so much stress on channelling and repressing sexual options, we'd all experience frequent lesser or greater shifts in our object-choice. You only have to look at children, who go through a stage of being just sexual, full stop. The way society is structured, however, it's much easier to opt for one fixed identity or the other.

I get very angry about the way bisexuals are characterized as perpetual Peter Pans, emotionally immature because we won't 'decide'. Why, I wonder, is it regarded as a sign of maturity to narrow your sexual potential? Might it not be immature to jettison a whole area of yourself, and a whole area in which you could relate to people, for the sake of acceptance into one of the two camps?

This often seems to be what it's about: the need, whether through unease or laziness, of others to be able to relate to us within clear-cut parameters. It's good that bisexuals are fighting back a bit now, for example by using the word 'monosexual' to describe those who are attracted to just one sex, whether their own or the opposite. Monosexuals have always used the bisexual's ability to have sexual relationships with either sex as a kind of insult, and now we're turning that around by suggesting that to confine yourself to just one sex is a reductive, limiting way of relating to people.

Another done-to-death stereotype is the 'promiscuous' bisexual. It seems to date from the swinging 60s, when a lot of people were experimenting sexually and bisexuals were seen as even less discriminating than the rest, with more sexual partners. The mood of the time encouraged people to be open about their experimentation, with the result that many essentially heterosexual people identified as bisexual when ultimately, or certainly long term, they were not.

The myth of the promiscuous bisexual was finally refuted for me after a conversation I had with a mixed group of older bisexuals in their forties and fifties. They maintained that overall they had had *fewer* sexual relationships than lesbian, gay or straight friends because for them relations with both sexes were 'less heightened, easier and more normalized'. They argued that if you're monosexual and meet a member of the sex you acknowledge being attracted to, there's always a moment, however brief, when you consider whether you're attracted to that individual or not. If you're bisexual, however, there isn't the same subdivision of new acquaintances, and because theoretically you could relate sexually to anyone, the sexual tension recedes and isn't such a feature of the way you relate to people in the early stages. A man in the group said, 'It's because there isn't a group that's outlawed to you, and there's no preferred group, so it stops being immediately important. It takes its place alongside a lot of other things, and when attraction happens it often happens later on, when I know somebody well.' In my own experience, I've found that I relate to women and men in much the same way, and seem to have fewer friendships that become sexual than some of my heterosexual friends.

I find I meet as much prejudice from the lesbian and gay community as from straight society. I'm sorry if that sounds like whingeing, but that's been my experience. Responses are often dismissive: as a bisexual you're regarded as being at one of the stages along the route to becoming fully lesbian or gay. While this may be true for some people, it certainly isn't for all. Often the result is that bisexuals submerge their 'het' side and give the people what they want. It's hardly surprising that people say they don't know many 'genuine bisexuals'.

Stories abound of lesbians and gays who have been 'burned' by having relationships with bisexuals who have 'reverted' to being straight. While the hurt caused by this situation can be enormous, I'm inclined to feel that too much emphasis on the possibility creates worse problems, discouraging women who begin to feel attracted to other women from acting in case they discover that they're wrong and have to face the accusations of playing fast and loose with a 'sister's' affections. I'd argue that for every woman acting cavalierly, there are ten who are being ultra-cautious, suppressing their feelings and staying firmly within heterosexual boundaries. Condemnation from lesbian sisters is the last thing potentially bisexual women need. Ultimately, this condemnation allies itself with reactionary opinion which preaches 'don't experiment, don't trust your own feelings, stay where you are'. It must be tremendously reassuring to advocates of the current right-wing backlash to find such controlling mechanisms coming from women themselves.

I should say that I *do* take on board the genuine criticism by separatist lesbians of bisexual women who are, as they see it, traitors colluding with the enemy. This is a valid political point of view. Less valid are the misogynist attitudes of sections of the gay scene, which can make a bisexual man's life far from pleasant.

Obviously bisexuals are not oppressed in the same way as lesbians and gays – bisexuals don't have their lives stigmatized to the same extent, are not as likely to be beaten up, and can always shuffle back to the safety of the straight world if things get too hot. If you plan on being openly lesbian or gay you can expect regular harassment, constant attacks on your sexuality, the loss of many of the personal and career expectations that being a nice, straight member of a nuclear family will get you. Let's face it, it's a good way of keeping a lot of waverers in line!

Straight society can distance itself from lesbians and gays: it can view them as totally 'other' and feel free to attack and distort the facts as much as it wants. Its attitude to bisexuals is more difficult, however, because here are people who *can*, if they choose, relate to the sex they're supposed to fancy. Bisexuality is threatening because bisexuals refute the idea of the 'naturalness' of heterosexuality and consequently of the 'unnaturalness' of homosexuality. Faced with this blurring of divisions, society doesn't rake up hate and disgust as it does with lesbians and gays; instead it copes with bisexuality by treating it as a bit of a joke and *refusing to take it seriously*. I consider this a mark of how disturbing society finds bisexuality. There's a certain air of desperation about it.

The frustration and lack of self-respect that goes with seeing their sexuality trivialized proves too much for many bisexuals, and after a few years they rush headlong into one of the two camps.

All that I've written might suggest a fairly pessimistic outlook for bisexuals, but I don't feel this to be the case. Whatever the disadvantages, politically and personally, the positive feeling I have that on several occasions I've come close to having a relationship with an *individual*, rather than with a member of a gender, makes it worthwhile. Maybe that's because I see more similarities than differences in male and female physiognomy, and find that I don't make love very differently with either sex. Yes, despite gender stereotyping ...

I find I have less sex now than when I was younger, and feel this is the same for most people, whether lesbian or gay, heterosexual or bisexual. Now I make love only when I know it's making love I really want, and not comfort, security, recognition in my work... It's easy when you're younger to feel a kind of unfocused need, and assume it's sex that you want. Later, you can differentiate, or at least most of the time! I enjoy meeting new women and men, maybe fancying them, maybe not. I enjoy having the freedom to muse about it and then, more often than not, leave it at that.

Respect
B. J. Addison

'Momma, why does a well-dressed white man ask a kid like me where he can find a nice black woman?'

I overheard my little brother ask this question one night when he came home from his part-time job in Greenwich Village. I was about twenty at the time and wondered how little brother got to be so naive, when every black female with half a brain knew that she had to go about as though she was entirely above reproach just in order to avoid having white men think she was 'that kind of woman'. What kind of woman? Why, the kind of woman a white stranger would ask a little kid for: an easy, sexy, hip-swinging woman who would be his for the asking, who would smile at his insensitivity, who would give him sex and who would never ask for anything, not anything. The kind of woman white men invented.

Of course, most white men simply assumed that any black female, regardless of age, was 'that kind of woman' — that's how it is when you become the victim of your own propaganda. This was the US in the 1950s, but having lived in Britain for over a decade I now realize that there are more similarities than I at first recognized. Attitudes haven't changed so much as gone underground.

The subject of black women and their sexuality was something I had not given much thought to for most of my life. More thought was given over to racism's squeaky wheel, and in fact it is racism that has shaped the sexuality of black women since they left Africa. Before then, black women (and men) could think of themselves as king, queen, soldier, artisan, sometimes, if captured in war, as slave. It is easy to romanticize life before the white man, especially as what came after has had little beauty. Yet as I have discovered more and more about our history I have learned that there is enough evidence to tell us that in the ancient world the black woman was worshipped as a goddess. There were black Madonnas all over Europe before the onset of Christianity, and many Christian temples were built over these shrines. In Africa great queens ruled, fought wars and made decisions that changed the lives of their people. To name but one, Dahia-al-Kahina of Mauritania drove an Arab army into Tripolitania. She was fierce, and when in retreat pioneered the 'scorched earth' tactic of destroying anything the enemy could use for food or shelter. It is hard to think of women like these as victims.

But when cunning, strength and ingenuity proved no match for gunpowder, when Africa lost control over her economy and was robbed of 60 million of her people at their highest level of productivity, her men and women lost control of the shape their sexuality could take, and more. Women have always been considered legitimate spoils of war, but slavery was not war, it was just a commercial enterprise, with human beings as its chief commodity. Black women were bought and sold like pieces of meat and forced to breed like animals. Black woman sacrificed her privacy and dignity to the auction block and her sexuality to those who bartered her life and the lives of her children and then forced her to have sex with them and then called her a slut for doing so.

Picture a cattle market. Eager buyers crowd around; they pull the cow's tail, stroke its flanks, lift its hooves, examine teeth, poke its private parts and speculate on the possible number of progeny. This is how our sexuality was (re)formed in the new world. What does sexuality matter to an animal without a soul? Why does a white man behave towards a decent black woman in a way he would never think of behaving towards any white woman?

The experience of black women in the US is similar enough to that of other black women of the diaspora to make comparisons. Black women, especially of an older generation, have many stories to tell about sexual exploitation, whether the sexual harassment they suffered in the rag trade in New York in the days of labour-intensive manufacturing – just part of the job, no different from slavery really – or in service in private houses throughout Europe and the US. Legions of black women worked as maids or cleaners, lived in or out, cooked, cleaned, were entrusted with the care of children, and in many cases were expected to have sex with the master of the house. But these women would never have been allowed to eat in the same restaurant as that man. I remember when I was ten or eleven years old listening to my mother and her friends talking about friends and relations who were 'in service'. It seemed to me then that if you were black and female, you were born with a broom in your hand. The word 'sex' was never used; they just talked about the master's 'overtures' to the cook or the maid, especially if she was young or pretty. She was ripe picking. Things were even worse in the deep south, where, by law, a black woman 'could not be raped', but if a black man so much as 'looked' at a white woman he could pay for it with his life. White women seem on the surface to have had a better deal, yet I sometimes wonder what it did to their sexuality too – how must it have felt to see your husband cohabiting and producing children with an 'inferior' black woman? The white woman had to grin and bear it, but it was not a choice over which she had any control either.

I grew up in the age of feminism; I was educated and progressive. I was also black. My sophisticated self said 'this is a great movement'; my black self said, 'what do these people have to offer me?' I remember feeling hostility, anger, sometimes a deep confusion. After all, black women had always worked, and not for careers, but out of need. They fought racism day and night, at their jobs, in the supermarket, everywhere. No black women in my experience sat around in groups discussing whether or not they had had an orgasm. Talking about sex was considered common and only for white folks: black sexuality had a different shape.

I went to a Catholic school, where virginity until marriage or death was the accepted standard. Growing up Roman Catholic in a racist and sexist society is a punishment, believe me – it inhibits warmth and spontaneity in favour of a constant awareness of 'being a good girl'. Sexuality to me meant not being pregnant before you were married. Our mothers feared that we would fall into the povery pit if we started producing children early, and they were right to warn us against it. I was never told anything specific about sex; it was more that we sensed a sad disapproval in the voices of elders when they talked about girls who had babies without being married, though these girls were hardly ever turned out and often their mothers looked after the children. I never knew the details of childbirth either until I was quite grown – we girls talked, but we didn't know the intricacies.

My mother was a social worker for the Church. Her job took her, and me, into the homes of black families who lived in tenement housing, always on the breadline, so I soon got to know what babies were – and not from dolls in my Christmas stocking. As a result I came to believe in birth control, despite the opinions of the Church. Though I am very fond of my friends' children, I have made a conscious choice not to have children myself – after all, you give at least eighteen years of your life to a child. It's a long time.

Unlike today we were not expected always to be thinking about sex – there was school and church and lots of activities. We went out mostly in mixed groups of boys and girls, so I had plenty of male company. When we started dating, at the age of fifteen or sixteen, our parents would want to know all about the boy and it was accepted that he would respect us and not try anything on. I remember when I was in college a neighbour of mine, a nice guy from a good family, wanting to have sex and telling me it was 'healthy'. I told my girlfriends and we laughed and laughed – yes, girls would get together and talk about boys, but we knew we would never let them try anything, even getting too close while dancing. We were 'nice' kids who didn't get into trouble. Restrictions were imposed by both Mother and Mother Church.

When I talk to women now about their adolescence and early adulthood I realize how constrained we were. It was not until I was in my twenties, in Europe, that I allowed myself to have sex for the first time. By then I was bored with the idea of my virginity and it seemed right to lose it. Far from home, I realized that I had to be responsible to myself, not to the Church, to my parents or to society. There was no romance – neither of us felt seriously about it. But you have to start somewhere.

So I grew up relatively ignorant but happy, despite the pressures. I was determined not to get married, but to have a career. I saw marriage as working mainly for the benefit of men and didn't believe women got a lot from it. Black girls grow up surrounded by experiences of women who have been left to bring up children on their own, so they know that marriage is no guarantee of anything. And even good men often cannot find work because of racism, so it's the woman who has to support the household. Black women are used to accommodating their sexuality to their situation; we didn't expect to be taken care of, having learned from bitter experience. That's our history. White women are more likely to expect to be looked after as a right, so they are often shocked when men leave them. As black women, we are likely to be sad rather than shocked or unable to carry on.

I believe the marriage 'norm' is too rigid. I don't think marriage is for everyone. Even in my early twenties I imagined a different kind of relationship – I used to say I wouldn't mind being married, as long as I didn't have to live with him. Once you realize marriage is not the only option, relationships become easier and you learn to trust your instincts about people rather than looking for a preconceived ideal. I like men – black and white – but though I have had several long and satisfying relationships, I have met few men I have wanted to spend all my time with. Part of me is suspicious of 'serious' relationships; I believe they stifle women and I find myself wary of becoming trapped. Once you cut out all the adolescent conditioning and media-generated needs, happiness can be found just as easily in work, supportive friends, someone to share your feelings with.

Sexuality to me is more all-encompassing than sex and has to do with a giving of the whole being. Sex is smaller and more limited and is involved with taking. To me, sexuality is an ever-present shadow; it's a kind of feeling that surfaces. I think it is something that black women always have but do not always acknowledge. After all, we are constantly being told how 'wanton' we are. I remember even as a child wondering why people who denigrated us publicly as loose or immoral would take advantage of us sexually in private at the first opportunity. This kind of ambivalence creates doubts deep inside about what kind of woman you will be; it's all these things that prevent your personality from having full flow. You find yourself reacting to negative expectations, not positive ones: 'don't wear loud colours', 'don't talk too loud', 'don't laugh too loud' ... otherwise 'people will think you're like those no account niggers'. My mother and black mothers through the ages have warned their daughters that whereas a man can roll around drunk in the gutter then change his shirt and be respectable again next day, a woman who does the same is damned forever, and a black woman forever and a day. All this is the dough out of which my sexuality has been shaped.

In retrospect, I can see that my parents, like other good black parents, tried to bring us up to be 'respectable', though not in a hard, cold, penny-pinching Victorian way. It was more that they worked hard to educate us so we could have an easier life than they had had; they were always afraid that we might slip back and so they pushed, gently and with humour. Though not a Catholic himself, my father always saw to it that we attended Mass and had everything we needed for school. They were good people and always there for me, and in this I consider myself fortunate – more so than some of my middle-class friends who have ended up on the psychiatrist's couch. We were graduates of the 'do as I say and not as I do' school.

When I talk to black women friends some say that when they were children they longed to be white. Really they wanted an easier life, which they perceived as possible only by being white. I can sympathize with these feelings; I was one of only three black children in my primary school, and in my Catholic high school one of perhaps six, all girls. That presented problems in adolescence: I remember having crushes on white boys – sometimes it was mutual, but neither of us would know what to do about it. We did know that we had to observe the conventions, however.

Through my adolescence my best girlfiend was also a church member. We hung out together all the time, mostly at her house. We exchanged Christmas and birthday presents, compared notes on our latest crushes, giggled a lot, studied, went to church affairs, sang in the church choir, and, of course, went to the movies and to the Apollo in Harlem. They were fun, those years, running through the subway to catch a train to 125th Street to the Apollo to see someone who is now a legend, going to high school dances, laughing, going to the prom when I was in college, joining the NAACP. Our sexuality just had to catch up as we went along.

We lived in the movies. Every Sunday after twelve o'clock Mass we would buy a bag of cakes and sit there all day, then back to my friend's house for dinner and home by nine or my mother would be on the phone asking where I was. Of course, we dreamed of the romantic love we saw depicted on screen – a nice man walking with his arm around your waist, a nice house – even though black women were never portrayed in that way.

Both my friend and her sister were beautiful girls; they looked like you were supposed to look in those days: long hair, aquiline noses, light skin. I felt like an ugly duckling – boys jumped over me to get to them. I also found that many black guys didn't like me because I was 'too intellectual'. University turned out to be the equalizer – they left to get married and I stayed on. Though we laughed about racism and tried to do our best, we always knew there were neighbourhoods we couldn't live in, jobs we would never be given, restaurants we couldn't eat in – and men we couldn't have. A black woman could lose her reputation by being seen with a white man (unless he was a priest) because everyone would assume that he only wanted her for sex. Yet despite those taboos, interracial couples did meet and forge loving relationships. And I've found in my own life I've always had relationships with white men, though not out of any deliberate aim – it's just happened that way.

In the days before black was beautiful a black person, no matter how well educated, could never expect to be evaluated according to his or her talents, intelligence or general grooming – in other words, as white people are. Black people used to joke if they were turned down for a job: 'well, they must have their quota for this week'. When I started work as a high-school graduate there were offices in which black people had never worked. Sometimes they would take on just two or three to test the reaction. Often recruitment organizations would screen applicants before they were let loose on a prospective employer – you would think you were being scrutinized for the job of Vice-president, or the Pope. It happened to me when I wanted to become an airline stewardess; I'm still waiting to hear the results.

Once I started work I encountered a more insidious form of racism. The white girls in the office were always friendly; we'd go for lunch and chat about who we thought was 'cute' and so on. They probably never intended to be racist, but though they themselves all wanted to go out with doctors or lawyers, they would bend over backwards to point out to me how 'cute' the elevator man was. I've nothing against elevator men, but I resented the fact that they assumed that I would not, like them, aspire to marry a man with a profession. It was as though these white women, fed with more positive images, automatically thought of themselves as 'better' and more privileged, no matter if they were less talented, less educated or even less attractive.

So I feel that black women's sexuality has always been soiled and distorted. Aretha sings of 'Respect', but where's the respect when a black academic is directed to the service elevator when she enters a 5th Avenue apartment for a dinner party? Or when a beautiful and talented performer like Lena Horne describes in her autobiography the humiliation of not being able to enter a hotel or club where she is performing by the front door? I can well remember as a child feeling uncomfortable when a tradesman called my mother by her first name, showing a familiarity he would never show to a white woman. Or when my aunt complained to a white man, a southerner, who had pushed in front of her in the taxi queue, and his reponse was: 'I know what I'd do if I had you down where I come from.' I always resented the time black women wasted trying to avoid situations in which they might be insulted or humiliated by white people.

I believe a negative image of black women is fostered by the media, which can't decide whether it wants us to be fat and shiny, or tall, sexy and smiling. Black women are possessed with a warmth and strength that is far removed from the images that appear in *Playboy* or the hysterical cackling creatures of most TV shows, all teeth and rolling eyes. The media has always separated good women from bad, and most roles available for black actressess fall into the bad woman stereotype: drug addicts, prostitutes, the sexy black wench. How can a young black woman's sexuality be developed positively when she sees reflected in the media only this type of image? Of course, the way white women are portrayed is also a distortion: no woman has the choice of how she's represented. But some women, white women, are lucky to be assigned less objectionable stereotypes.

It takes a long time to shake off the old taboos, but it can be done. When I was a young girl, what I wanted most was to be a woman. I thought that only then would I be happy. I believed this could only happen away from the country I was brought up in, and certainly it was not until I came to Europe that I began to put all this into perspective.

I believe now that perhaps it will be possible for black women to change, to reshape our sexuality and take it into a new era. This has implications for both men and women: men must stop excusing themselves for the things they do to women, and women must raise male children who are strong enough to reject peer pressure. Feminism has helped a great deal; it has enabled both black and white women to begin to define the questions and elaborate on the answers. And perhaps helping white women to face their own oppression will also help them to see the dimensions of ours.

For now, I am not sure what happiness means. Just like everyone else I've had my traumas and heartbreaks, but I'm alive, healthy, supported by loving friends who are my surrogate family. I look forward to the future with anticipation. I'm a fighter and a survivor. I'm a black woman.

I want the world to shift on its axis
Marie McShea

I am a lesbian. I believe passionately in my right to love women with my heart, my soul and my body. My sexual identity is a basic part of my life. It informs how I view the world and how the world looks at me. It is both political and personal. I am a sexual being. I want to make love, and be made love to. I want the world to shift on its axis from time to time, I want to be able to explore how this happens.

I haven't always been so open and confident. I emerged from childhood with my sexuality tightly bound up, and an implicit belief that sex was dirty. It has taken years of hard and often painful work to let go of my beliefs. I have been motivated by the recognition that sex could be exciting, by one particularly loving and challenging partner, and in recent years by my experience as a mother.

In consciously choosing to have a child I vowed to avoid the mistakes of my own childhood. I wanted my daughter to grow up confident and open about herself. And yet, as I live through her childhood there have been so many parallels with my own, I feel I have little choice but to continue to unravel my own experiences, to understand them, and work for change.

I confess to finding the exploration of my sexual identity difficult at times. I have felt embarrassed and lacking in confidence to talk openly. I have felt the words rise high above me and emblazon themselves in neon lights. I have felt the world watching and judging. Part of this is to do with my own vulnerability, but part is from the resounding silence around our sexuality. Speaking out about what we do in bed and who we do it with is taboo. And yet, I believe that if we break the silence and talk of who and how we are, it creates a wider picture of the many choices we can make. We discover we are not alone and we can feel better about ourselves. Also, more selfishly, I find that talking out the processes gives me a strength and distance to make resolution.

And so ... back to my beginnings ... the time, the 1950s, the place, Sydney, Australia.

My father died when I was eighteen months, leaving my mother a widow in her late thirties, a son of fourteen, and me. After what was no doubt a reasonable period of mourning and adjustment, my mother began to have sexual relationships. She 'chose' not to find a good man to marry and settle down with. Instead there was a succession of boyfriends who stayed for periods of between six months and six years. My memory (actually affirmed by my adult perception) says that the better ones were already married to someone else, and the others were weak and humourless. The mixture of clandestine affairs and boring outings left me feeling uncomfortable at the very least. I hated the change in my mother's behaviour when her lovers were around. She would give power away to them, wait on their needs, smile excitedly (or politely) at their jokes and stories, and change plans at a single phonecall. I was aware of a charged physicality. They were discreet in my presence but I have memories of heavy breathing and muffled groans in the dark after I had supposedly gone to sleep.

In retrospect, the adult in me can understand more clearly my mother's choices. She enjoyed relationships and did not want, at thirty-nine, to bury her sexuality with my father. After years of shame on my part, I am beginning to admire her courage in not giving in to societal conventions. But my reaction at the time was to dislike the men and hate the evidence of sexual activity in my mother. No one talked to me about what was happening, and my mother didn't give me any context for her desire for relationships. I just knew that she and I were living outside the conventional family of father, mother and children that all my friends seemed to have, and that was reflected in the books and films of the time. Also, importantly for me, lack of information meant that I found the entrances and exits of these men in my life unpredictable. I was frequently left with her friends or my grandmother with little or no warning ... the age-old problem of childcare.

The negative feeling about my mother's sexuality was reinforced by my brother who, I have subsequently discovered, condemned my mother as a 'damned whore'. While I can't recall any comments from the time, I knew by his silences, his body language and his early departure from home around sixteen or seventeen, that he thought my mother was wanton and amoral.

The result was that I took on board an unquestioned and questioning view that sex was unclean, if not dirty. I was afraid of desire and passion. I was afraid of what the pantings and the groans meant.

Pleasure in my own body was halted abruptly:

I am around six or seven ... I can remember very clearly a warm summer's morning ... it was around six-thirty ... and I'd evolved a complex system of masturbation, lying on my front against my thumbs. I'd assumed my mother was asleep and was shocked when she appeared beside my bed demanding to know what I was doing. Despite my silence (I didn't know what I was doing), she knew, and made it very clear that what I was doing was bad, and I should never do it again.

In the general atmosphere of denial and censure I didn't twiddle another thumb for over fifteen years until, in the context of early feminism, I discovered that it was 'normal' after all.

A residual curiosity was cut off at age nine. My friend Angela and I had mutually explored one another's bodies under the guise of a game called doctors and nurses. In the interest of science we maintained a record of crude autographed pictures. Naively I kept them in my ten-way purse. I forgot about them until I lost the purse at school one day, a day my friend Angela was sick. I remember being kept in after school and lectured in a high moral tone that nice girls didn't do things like this. The teacher, no doubt well meaning, told me that what I had done was dirty and that I should be ashamed of myself. She succeeded ... I was ashamed. My guilt was reinforced by the fact that Angela for some reason escaped censure.

Until very recently I assumed that repression was the basis for my fears and my closed-down state. But I discovered in writing this article a further piece of the puzzle:

> I am around seven ... eight. His name is Joe. There have already been a few before him. He is not married. He flies planes. He is a strong man.
>
> It's night. I waken from sleep. It's dark. I can't see much. I hear muffled sounds. I call out, 'Mummy ... Mummy'. No one comes. I get up ... walk towards sounds in the other bedroom. It sounds like whispering.
>
> It seems so very dark. I am afraid.
> I hear her saying no ... no ... no.
> I can't move. I can't see anything. I feel her fear.
> The picture goes blank.
> I go back to bed.
> I cry myself to sleep.

We never spoke about that incident, not in any of the years before her death the year I was twenty-eight. We each chose to deal with what had happened in different ways. In my memory she continued to go out with him. I suspect I blamed her for that. As for me, I'd witnessed my mother forced into something, and though I blocked it out I was left with an unacknowledged fear. A fear of sexual desire.

I was afraid of the power of another person's desire. I carried the fear around, unprocessed, into my early thirties. It was untouched by my early sexual encounters, and kept my responses to myself. I dampened my desires *and* encouraged my partners to do likewise. I didn't close off my sexuality, I just kept deeper responses tightly contained. My first orgasms happened in total silence. I was unwilling to make myself vulnerable to my partners.

In my early twenties I had two relationships of three years apiece, both with men. My desire melted a chink in my armour in the early months – I wanted and was wanted. However my fears and inability to trust soon cooled everything down. I gradually closed up again. I remember held-on-to orgasms in the foreplay and a faked enthusiasm about coming. Inside the joint filters of self-repression and what was in reality lack of interest in men, it didn't occur to me that my sexual responses were protected. What I didn't name to myself and didn't talk about, I didn't miss. The irony was that the times were said to be sexually permissive and I thought I was as well. I equated sexual liberation with the number of partners I had been with. Between my two long-term relationships I slept with a number of different boys.

I did have an active fantasy life around women and older girls. At ten I dreamt of various sports mistresses whisking me off over the horizon. In adolescence my imaginings became more physical, extending to kissing, cuddling and sharing a bed. I had chronic crush symptoms, always wanting some particular girl to be close. At thirteen my mother put me in boarding school for a brief time and I remember stroking and being aroused by the girl I was sleeping next to. We barely spoke by day. There were several friendships with teachers which teetered on the line of intimacy.

I never named these responses and even when I went to bed with one of my closest friends (we were disturbed by her boyfriend who awoke from his drunken stupor) I didn't recognize my lesbianism.

Retrospectively I can see there was a surreptitious stripping of bits of the armour and certainly with women I wanted to open up. But my confidence to initiate and sustain a sexual relationship didn't develop until I was twenty-six, when I finally brought my fantasies into alignment with a real relationship. My self-repression however did not suddenly disappear. I may have taken off the coat of chain-mail but I kept on the undergarments. With one woman lover sex was more like mutual masturbation. We aroused each other to gentle orgasm by clitoral stimulation with fingers and tongues. We read together books such as *Loving Women* and *The Joy of Lesbian Sex* which I seem to remember reinforced this 'nice' picture. While I found an enjoyment I'd never felt with men, I was restrained – my orgasms were quiet and centred in my clitoris. I never came loudly, never came groaning and shuddering with overwhelming satisfaction. Neither did she.

At the time I didn't know I was repressing my responses. I didn't know I was holding on to fear. I didn't know there was a vast space of abandonment and letting go. I have an image of myself swaddled in bandages. As each layer came off I felt lighter and freer, but I never knew how many layers there were 'protecting' and restraining me.

When I was thirty a woman came along who wanted more. She aroused a louder passion in me and offered a breadth of sexuality I had not experienced. Unaware of my fears and repression, I responded with the desire I felt. Difficulties arose however because suddenly I unconsciously came face to face with the sexuality I had condemned in my mother. I felt sexual. I was being sexual. I was letting go. Desire was suddenly unfettered and I was scared. I was feeling the very things I'd been ashamed of in my mother. My desire was dampened again. It first came to the surface around penetration. I had concurred and then suddenly froze as her fingers entered me. At the time I didn't understand why, and my first response was to deny any fear. Through her support I was able to move past my fear of penetration itself, but it took a long time to make connections.

Within the security of that relationship I began to process my childhood experiences. Until then they were unfiled. But it was a slow process and the effect on the relationship was marked. My sexual responses were unpredictable and misleading through my lack of insight. As a result our sexual relationship was uneven, and while there were times when the earth moved, this was not a consistent reality. We stayed together for six years, both of us working and resolving and reworking many issues. At that point we chose to transform our close bond into a friendship. She is now my sister, my colleague, my friend, my daughter's co-parent, but no longer my lover.

Since then I have had other important sexual relationships and I've discovered how to revel more fully in my desires and to be proud of them. I've also learned how to examine my processes in general, and take greater responsibility for my feelings. I have learned to enjoy myself. I have learned to place the sexual responses I have had from childhood. I know now that those feelings about sex and sexuality were specific to then. These feelings have no relevance to my present life. I may have had to repress myself as a child, but I sure as hell don't have to now.

In owning my sexuality I become more and more interested in exploring further the boundaries of sexual desire. I am fascinated by the ways in which sexual tensions can be awakened and sustained, and how these work in lesbian relationships. I am excited by the tensions involved in initiating and holding the power of arousing a woman to come; as well as in completely giving up power and control to another in letting go. This is a long way from the nice sexuality embodied in my lesbian feminist framework of the 1970s. In the late 1980s and early 1990s in London there have been a number of passionate public discussions around desire and how to sustain it. The traditional models of 'butch' and 'femme' are being explored, with the recognition that there is much in these models that may be relevant today. For me this did not involve deciding that I am either butch or femme; rather I can recognize how I can use the sexual tension generated by those roles.

At present I am not in a relationship. But this is irrelevant to whether or not I am a sexual person. I have desires and can respond to women sexually. I am extremely cautious about entering a relationship until I have the knowledge, or courage to believe, that another woman is equally committed to the hard work involved in a good relationship.

But where does all this leave me as a mother?

My daughter's time and place are the 1990s in London, England. Yet as I said earlier, there are enough structural similarities with the environment in which I grew up for me to be very aware of the possibility of repeating some of the patterns.

Despite my intentions to the contrary, my daughter is being raised in what is essentially a single-parent context. She too has a sexually active mother, and in both instances the society outside condemns that sexuality. I took in messages as a child that my mother was wrong to have sexual relationships not sanctified by marriage. It is very possible that my daughter could take in similar messages because I too am outside the heterosexual norm.

Recognizing the similarities has pushed me towards a need to be clear to myself and to her about who I am. As so much of my childhood belief systems were born out of innuendo and silence, my prime commitment to my daughter is communication. I do slip up sometimes, but my goal is to give her as much information as she can handle, according to her maturity. Because her beginnings are tied up with my lesbianism, this has involved deciding how to explain the process of self-insemination. I wanted her to know that she could meet her father (which she has) but that she has no father in the social sense of the word. She does have a mother and a co-parent living 200 miles away who has given me and her much support since her birth. Perhaps because I feel resolved about that choice, and because we have always been clear, she has seemed at ease with day-to-day living.

Within her growing complexity of understanding she has always known that we are lesbians. But from time to time she questions the meaning. Nearly two years ago at a Clause 28 demonstration, in her own process of learning to read she asked what was a 'l..e..s..b..i..a..n'. Silence seemed to descend around us as people awaited my reply to a six year old. I answered that it was a woman whose closest person was another woman. I compared it to her best friend's mother and stepfather who are similarly close. I am still happy with this definition and trust I will be able to expand it to include a sexual dimension when this is appropriate.

Being open does put some weight on her. On my part I want her to know that I have the right to acknowledge my sexuality. But in letting her know this I am aware that I need to protect her from subtle and overt projections which come her way because her mother is known as a lesbian. I have had to tell her that she may need to be careful who she talks to about it, struggling in the morass that comes from her questions as to why some people believe lesbianism is wrong.

In view of my own experiences of my mother's sexuality, I have been afraid my daughter may be shocked by evidence of my own. While I do not restrain myself from outward shows of affection – I will kiss or hug my lovers – I catch myself stifling desire until she is well asleep, and then keeping a vague ear out. I do not want to find ways of explaining sexual practice at this time. I recognize this is a dilemma for all sexually active parents, but I do feel the added weight of my lesbianism.

In terms of her own sense of her sexual identity I want her to feel free to make her own choices about who she relates to sexually, and how she does that. At present she is an extremely gregarious child and that feels positive. But I take each day as it comes.

Ultimately I have to trust in my ability to make the appropriate decisions, and to operate with foresight. I am fortunate in the choices I have made in my life that have led me to a place where I have the confidence to question my sexual responses and my sexual history. I am also fortunate in having a support system of friends and a political context with other lesbians that reflects an underlying validity for my choices. This good fortune is tempered though by an awareness of how isolated my mother was during the 1950s. She had different choices and little support. I believe now that she did the best she could. I respect her finally. I am glad she enjoyed her sexuality. I trust her granddaughter, like me, will too.

Acknowledgements

We dedicate this book to each and every contributor, in heartfelt appreciation of their honesty, integrity and willingness to uncover their lives.

Now, with this book almost in print, it seems a long time ago that we first began the work of seeking contributions from women and talking to them about the book we were planning.

There are women who have helped this book along the way, from conception to delivery, not only with a willingness to talk about their life experience, but in other ways as well.

We wish to thank Marie McShea for introducing us to three of the contributors and for making a significant contribution to the editing process of those articles. Thank you also to Judy Corbett for typing some of the first articles received and for doing some of the transcribing from tape.

When Scarlet Press decided to accept *Women Talk Sex*, their editors Christine Considine and Vicky Wilson were faced with a series of complex issues. Ought they to maintain a 'professional publisher's outlook', an outside position, or work with a more subjective understanding of the process and content? Their thoughtful sensitivity was as impressive as it was helpful, and their suggestions showed how clearly they understood our efforts and aims. The book has benefited from their skilful and caring editing and we thank them sincerely.

Patricia Duncker acccepted the task of writing an Introduction and we are grateful to her for contextualizing the content in a way that we three editors could not have done from our 'involved' position as editors and contributors.

Finally, we wish to thank all the women who began with the intention of writing for this book, whether by telling of their experience on tape, with written notes or in articles. Some of those contributions do not appear here, but they are no less a part of the history and process of this book's journey into the world.

Pearlie McNeill
Bea Freeman
Jenny Newman

Also from Scarlet Press

Women and Bisexuality
Sue George

Recent surveys show that approximately one-third of the population is bisexual, that is has sexual and emotional relationships with people of both genders. Yet despite a growing awareness of the fluidity of sexual desire and openness in talking about sex and sexual practice, no full-length book has analysed bisexuality with specific reference to women. In this pioneering study, Sue George examines the way bisexuality has been regarded or ignored by sexologists from the nineteenth century onwards and looks at how women who have relationships with people of both sexes construct their own identities and manage their lives.
ISBN 1 85727 072 1 pb / 1 85727 066 5 hb

Lesbians Talk Queer Notions
Cherry Smyth

Scarlet Press brings back the pamphlet as a forum for debate with the first in the **Lesbians Talk Issues** series – **Lesbians Talk Queer Notions.** What is this queer politics? Who are Queer Nation, OutRage, Act Up? Is there a queer aesthetic? And whose agenda is it anyway? Cherry Smyth discusses the implications of the new political radicalism with an international group of activists and their critics.
ISBN 1 85727 025 8

Lesbians Talk Safer Sex
Sue O'Sullivan and Pratibha Parmar

Is safer sex an issue for lesbians? Are lesbians and other women taken into account in current research on HIV transmission and treatment for Aids? What has the Aids crisis led us to discover about lesbian sexual practices and safer sexual practices? Sue O'Sullivan and Prathiba Parmar discuss the issues.
ISBN 1 85727 020 7